Pedro Encarnação, Sylvie Ray-Kaeser and Nicole Bianquin (Eds.)

GUIDELINES FOR SUPPORTING CHILDREN WITH DISABILITIES' PLAY. METHODOLOGIES, TOOLS, AND CONTEXTS.

This article/publication is based upon work from COST Action TD 1309
supported by COST (European Cooperation in Science and Technology).

COST (European Cooperation in Science and Technology) is a funding agency for research and innovation networks. Our Actions help connect research initiatives across Europe and enable scientists to grow their ideas by sharing them with their peers. This boosts their research, career and innovation

www.cost.eu

EUROPEAN COOPERATION IN SCIENCE & TECHNOLOGY

Funded by the Horizon 2020 Framework Programme of the European Union

Pedro Encarnação, Sylvie Ray-Kaeser
and Nicole Bianquin (Eds.)

GUIDELINES FOR SUPPORTING CHILDREN WITH DISABILITIES' PLAY.

METHODOLOGIES, TOOLS, AND CONTEXTS.

ISBN 978-3-11-061343-8
e-ISBN (PDF) 978-3-11-061344-5
e-ISBN (EPUB) 978-3-11-061372-8

Published by De Gruyter Poland Ltd, Warsaw/Berlin
Part of Walter de Gruyter GmbH, Berlin/Boston
The book is published with open access at www.degruyter.com.

Library of Congress Cataloging-in-Publication Data
A CIP catalog record for this book has been applied for at the Library of Congress.

www.degruyteropen.com

Cover illustration by Arianna, aged 7 years, entitled 'Swimming pool'
Drawings in pages 6, 27 and 84 were created by students of the Department of Graphic Design of the School of Applied Arts and Design, Zagreb, Croatia, under the mentorship of their teacher Tomislav Tomić, MA Graphic Arts.
Drawings in page 20, 23 and 66 were created by students of the St Edward's college, Malta, under the mentorship of their art teacher Lisa Pace.

Editors

Pedro Encarnação

Católica Lisbon School of Business & Economics

Universidade Católica Portuguesa

Lisbon, Portugal

Sylvie Ray-Kaeser

Occupational Therapy Department

School of Social Work and Health

University of Applied Sciences and Arts of Lausanne

Lausanne, Switzerland

Nicole Bianquin

Department of Human and Social Sciences

University of Aosta Valley

Aosta, Italy

Contributors

Chapter 1 – What is play?

Serenella Besio
Department of Human and Social Sciences
Università degli Studi di Bergamo
Bergamo, Italy

Chapter 2 – Do children with disabilities play?

Serenella Besio
Department of Human and Social Sciences
Università degli Studi di Bergamo
Bergamo, Italy

Vaska Stancheva-Popkostadinova
Department of Medical-Social Sciences
Faculty of Public Health, Health Care and Sports
South-West University 'Neofit Rilski'
Blagoevgrad, Bulgaria

Chapter 3 – What barriers to play do children with disabilities face?

Helen Lynch

Department of Occupational Science and Occupational Therapy

University College Cork

Cork, Ireland

Alice Moore

Department of Occupational Science and Occupational Therapy

University College Cork

Cork, Ireland

Chapter 4 – Are our children playing?

Daniela Bulgarelli

Department of Human and Social Sciences

University of Aosta Valley

Aosta, Italy

Francesca Caprino

INDIRE (National Institute for Documentation, Innovation and Educational Research)

Central Regional Unit

Rome, Italy

Chapter 5 – How can I, as an adult, facilitate play?

Nicole Bianquin

Department of Human and Social Sciences

University of Aosta Valley

Aosta, Italy

Chapter 6 – What Assistive Technologies exist to enable participation in play?

Pedro Encarnação

Católica Lisbon School of Business & Economics

Universidade Católica Portuguesa

Lisbon, Portugal

Rianne Jansens

Faculty of Health Care

Zuyd University of Applied Sciences

Heerlen, the Netherlands

Chapter 7 – Which toys and games are appropriate for our children?

Sylvie Ray-Kaeser

Occupational Therapy Department

School of Social Work and Health

University of Applied Sciences and Arts of Lausanne

Lausanne, Switzerland

Odile Perino
FM2J – Centre National de Formation aux Métiers du Jeu et du Jouet
Lyon, France

Maria Costa
AIJU – Technological Institute for Children's Products and Leisure
Alicante, Spain

Eleanor Schneider
Department of Occupational Therapy
University of Haifa
Haifa, Israel

Vardit Kindler
Dvorah Agmon Pre-School Development Center
Jerusalem, Israel

Andrea Bonarini
Department of Electronics, Information, and Bioengineering
Politecnico di Milano
Milan, Italy

Chapter 8 – Which digital games are appropriate for our children?

Agnieszka Landowska

Faculty of Electronics, Telecommunications and Informatics

Gdansk University of Technology

Gdansk, Poland

Chapter 9 – Which spaces are appropriate for our children?

Helen Lynch

Department of Occupational Science and Occupational Therapy

University College Cork

Cork, Ireland

Chapter 10 – Take home messages

Pedro Encarnação

Católica Lisbon School of Business & Economics

Universidade Católica Portuguesa

Lisbon, Portugal

Sylvie Ray-Kaeser

Occupational Therapy Department

School of Social Work and Health

University of Applied Sciences and Arts of Lausanne

Lausanne, Switzerland

Nicole Bianquin
Department of Human and Social Sciences
University of Aosta Valley
Aosta, Italy

Serenella Besio
Department of Human and Social Sciences
Università degli Studi di Bergamo
Bergamo, Italy

Table of Contents

Foreword

When thinking about children, one automatically thinks about play. Play is something which comes in different forms, elderly may think of play as something manual or traditional, whilst the younger generation will definitely think on the digital lines of play. Play has evolved through time and although sometimes we may feel irritated by the fact that manual play is lacking in today's world, we must admit that technology has stepped up play also due to the fact that now it is also targeting to become more accessible to everyone, including children with various forms of impairments.

The United Nations Convention on the Rights of the Child also mentions the right to play for every child in its Article 31. This strengthens the argument that play has to be offered to everyone, all children need to be included and have the chance to be creative, to physically participate and therefore have a harmonious cognitive development. We have to keep in mind that we have all been children and we know by fact that play, apart from entertaining us, helped us grow stronger and better because it gave us the opportunity to experience freedom, curiosity, imagination, etc. Play also develops concentration, a form of following rules (if the game has rules), repetition, planning, problem solving and satisfaction.

One doesn't play if playing that game or playing with that toy does not satisfy him or her, therefore play is also a matter of option. A child might like playing board games, others might like playing with other stuff which is not really meant to be toys such as, for example, a sauce pen (which might be considered as grown up stuff). There is another important facet in play, which is the social aspect. There are children that like playing with other children, sharing toys or playing a game together, and there are other children that prefer playing alone. It is known that play changes through childhood and children themselves change the way they look at play and the way they choose to play. A description of the different types of play and of play development through childhood can be found in Chapter 1 of this book.

In 2006, the World Health Organization (WHO), through the International Classification of Functioning, Disability and Health: Children and Youth Version, recognised play as an important factor for children wellbeing and health. It is a known fact that through ensuring equal opportunities in play, we are investing in having a more inclusive society. Through play children interact with each other and thus it is very important that play is accessible for all children, including all children with disabilities. However, it is still common that children with disabilities face barriers to play. I remember being a young child with physical disability (Spina Bifida) who loved playing with other children. I loved to participate in physical activities, such as playing football or taking part in games organized by the Scout group. Obviously I was faced with obstacles and my peers had to adapt the game to my needs, but when this was done it ended up creating an inclusive environment which not only myself as a disabled child, but also my friends who where creative enough to adapt the game to my needs, benefited from.

The 'Guidelines for Supporting Children with Disabilities' Play' developed by the COST Action 'LUDI - Play for Children with Disabilities' are essential for children themselves, parents (guardians) and all professionals working with children. The book highlights the importance of play for children, including those with disabilities, the barriers children with disabilities face in play, and how can an adult facilitate play. The guidelines also look at different assistive technologies that enable children with disabilities to participate in play and gives a deep insight on what type of games (including digital games), spaces/environments and toys are appropriate for children with disabilities.

In my opinion, as a professional working in the disability sector in Malta and also as a disabled person myself, I believe that such Guidelines are a valuable tool to raise awareness on the importance of play and I will certainly use them to advocate for children with disabilities play rights in Malta.

Oliver Scicluna
Commissioner for the Rights of Persons with Disability, Malta
LUDI Advisory Board member

Preface

Pedro Encarnação, Sylvie Ray-Kaeser and Nicole Bianquin

Play is a children's right, enshrined in several international conventions. Many research studies show how much play for the sake of play, i.e. play 'only' for recreational pleasure and fun, without any secondary goal, is important for children's wellbeing and development. However, in today's society, play is often considered unproductive and a waste of time. Children with disabilities in particular face many barriers to fully enjoy their right to play, including attitudinal, organizational or systemic, architectural or physical, and technological barriers.

Although play in general is an established research area and children with disabilities' play has been addressed by several studies, there is a lack of a multidisciplinary and integrated perspective on the theme, focusing on play for the sake of play. This called for the need of joining together physiatrists, physical therapists, occupational therapists, psychologists, pedagogists, childhood educators and teachers, assistive technology practitioners and developers, engineers, designers, architects, disability studies' scholars and activists, policy makers, young persons with disabilities and their significant ones to jointly address the subject of Play for Children with Disabilities.

COST is the longest-running European framework supporting trans-national cooperation among researchers, engineers and scholars across Europe. It funds pan-European networks, called 'COST Actions', of scientists and researchers across all science and technology fields. The COST Action TD1309 | Play for Children with Disabilities (LUDI) (2014-2018, www.ludi-network.eu | www.cost.eu/td1309) is a network involving more than 100 persons from 32 European countries, including all the groups listed above, working towards the creation of a novel and autonomous field of research and intervention on play for children with disabilities. Three main objectives were set for the COST Action LUDI:

a) Collecting and systematizing all existing competence and skills, such as educational researches, clinical initiatives, know-how of resources centres and users' associations;

b) Developing new knowledge related to settings, tools and methodologies associated with the play of children with disabilities; and

c) Disseminating the best practices emerging from the joint effort of researchers, practitioners and users.

Overall, LUDI aims at spreading awareness on the importance of giving children with disabilities the opportunity to play, ensuring equity in their exercise of the right to play, by putting play at the centre of the multidisciplinary research and intervention on children with disabilities.

This book encompasses all the work done within LUDI on play for children with disabilities. It aims to provide, in layperson's language, pragmatic, ready-to-use information for all of those interested in the theme, from scholars to parents looking for solutions on how to enable and support children with disabilities' play.

More specifically, the objectives of these 'Guidelines for supporting children with disabilities' play', are

a) Develop an understanding of what is play and its importance for child development (Chapter 1);

b) Identify specific play challenges in different disability groups (Chapter 2);

c) Raise awareness on play as a right for every child and on the barriers that children with disabilities may face when exercising their right to play (Chapter 3);

d) Provide tools for assessing children's play (Chapter 4);

e) Discuss methodologies for adults to facilitate children with disabilities' play (Chapter 5);

f) Guide adults when considering assistive technology to support play and when selecting toys, physical or digital games, or playspaces for their children (chapters 6 to 9);

g) List the key ideas around children with disabilities' play (Chapter 10); and

h) Enumerate a vast series of resources where one can find more information on play for children with disabilities (Chapters 11). Bibliographic references for the literal quotes included in the book can be found in this Chapter 11.

This publication was only possible thanks to each chapter's authors, which selflessly contributed with their work and expertise, willingly and patiently accommodating our comments and suggestions.

The book is also the result of the knowledge chaired within the LUDI network in several meetings, scientific conferences, short scientific visits, training schools and joint publications. Our gratitude goes to all LUDI members, LUDI Advisory Board members, international experts, policy makers, children with disabilities and their families that took part in these activities. We would also like to acknowledge the Università della Valle d'Aosta that hosted the Action, providing all the necessary administrative support, and COST that supported the LUDI network.

Finally yet importantly, we would like to thank all the children who made beautiful drawings to illustrate the book.

1

What is play?

Serenella Besio

Children are such stuff as plcy is made on

Play!

We all know what is meant when we talk about play. Indeed, everyone considers himself an expert in play, simply because we have been children and we have played. Not only do we know many types of play but above all, we know the feelings it produces: happiness, getting lost, suspension of reality, the absolute concentration in the most total lightness. We know also its contradictions, such as the essential need to respect the rules mixed with the most uncontrolled fantasy.

We experienced the joy of imagining without limits, of playing roles in the shoes of others, of building original environments with various materials, of launching one's body in a race or in a competition. We immediately recognise the gleam – pure life – in the gaze of a friend who invites us, without words, to play. There are no barriers or differences – social, geographical, ethnic, of gender or age – that can prevent children from playing; no translations or special interpretations are necessary for them to agree on how to play.

Adults often cultivate some forms of playful activities throughout their lives. But once in a while every adult cannot avoid answering to an impromptu proposal of play that comes from a child, that shows up in a day of vacation, that originates from a secret thought. Then, in a moment, the adult feels like a child again, and those sensations come back alive, real, unchanged over time. In some happy cases, that gleam in the eyes of those who accept or launch a playful provocation can also be encountered in an elderly person, reviving the liveliness of childhood time.

The origin of play is lost in the mists of time. It seems to belong to the human species since the very beginning. We can consider the primitives' paintings in the caves as a first expression of playfulness, as well as their use of propitiatory masks highlighted in the rock engravings (dating up to 30,000 years ago). It is worth to remember that the oldest known toy – a parallelepiped in clay with round recesses – was found in Bulgaria, dating back to the 5th millennium BC. Toys were usually buried in children's graves among the Sumerians, the Egyptians, the Greeks and the Romans. The awareness that other animal species play – mammals, birds, but also reptiles and insects – is another proof in favour of the hypothesis that play is an innate competence. How can we be sure? We know this because we recognise play when it is there, and we can also describe it in these animals, for some typical characteristics, including the manifestation of pleasure, gratuity, the correlation with the absence of concomitant vital and stressing activities (hunting, feeding, sleeping, ...)

But what is play then? How can it be defined? Western culture has been dealing with this question since its origins, under many perspectives: philosophy, from Plato onwards, along the history of its pedagogical branch, through Locke, Fénelon, Fröbel, Montessori, Dewey; psychology, with the main contributions of its leading representatives in the study of childhood (Piaget, Vygotskij, Bruner, Winnicott), and the scholars that followed, up to today (Smilansky, Rubin, Garvey, Santrock, Parten); ethology, with Tinbergen first and Burghardt in our days. Among the most brilliant and fruitful interpretations, however, are those of scholars who – adopting a playful and irreverent approach – have overcome the rigid boundaries between the traditional disciplines. Johan Huizinga studied the play as a necessary foundation for culture and social organisation, in such an original way that he gave new significance to cultural anthropology. The eclectic Gregory Bateson offered the idea, very fruitful both for scientific speculation and for educational applications, of play as a 'frame', as a diverse world. Roger Caillois established the most original and inventive classification for all the forms of play into four categories – agon, alea, mimicry and ilinx. Brian Sutton-Smith, an excellent and prolific scholar in the field, has succeeded in establishing the play as a discipline in its own right.

It is therefore not surprising that the literature on play is very wide and has explored the most diverse perspectives, so as to identify and describe many features. In contrast to this wealth of reflections, however, there is an astonishing evidence: in fact, the scholars have not found, over time, an agreement on a single definition of the phenomenon. Indeed, Sutton-Smith himself, after an umpteenth review of studies on the subject, declared that 'no single definition could contain it'. And if this finding can, on the one hand, freshen the enthusiasm of those who exalt the elusiveness and the mystery of play, on the other, as Burghardt has effectively argued, it challenges the scientific validity of different play studies. Without a shared definition it is not possible to compare results, to test hypothesis, to identify research lines or assess the progress in the knowledge on play.

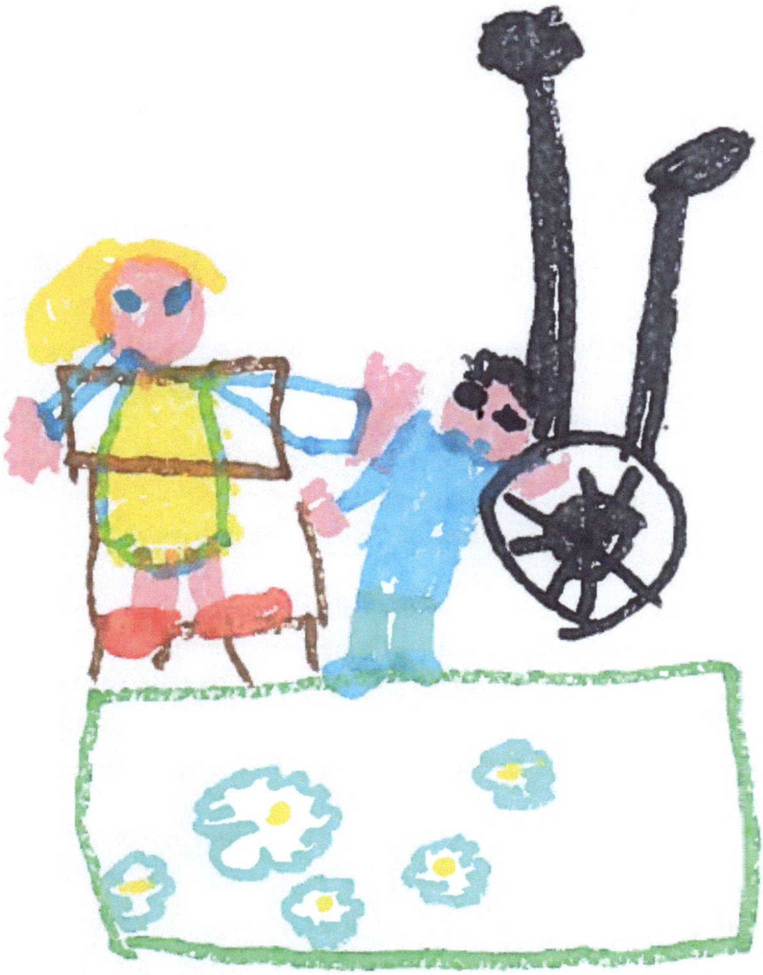

Beatrice, 5 years old, Italy

Definition and fundamentals of play

LUDI adopted Garvey's 1990 definition of play: 'Play is a range of voluntary, intrinsically motivated activities associated with recreational pleasure and enjoyment'. Among the many characteristics of play described in the literature, some of them are worthy of mention:

- a feeling of *freedom* is related to play, that players deeply perceive and can also be recognized by people observing others playing; a freedom which is neither disorder nor laziness;

- *pleasure* and/or fun are always associated to play too, to the point that they have been considered as an unavoidable dimension of play and are today considered as a value in themselves;

- play requires and claims for *concentration, intensity, seriousness* - we all know how difficult is to detach a child from his/her toy or to interrupt the game of a group of children; the play activity is immersive and an absent-minded play companion is immediately scolded by his/her peers;

- play is the main way through which children reveal their inexhaustible willingness to take active part in the life of their environment; it is in fact driven by *intrinsic* motivation – the new-born shows an immediate interest into playful interactions with the adult, children are naturally and constantly oriented towards play, etc.; by curiosity – to explore how a tool may be used, to experiment new rules of a game, etc.; by surprise – which often is the key to start playing; and also by challenge – to find a solution to a problem in a board or a construction game, to set difficult goals or to impose new constraints to make a game more complex, etc.

Six aspects, called 'fundamentals of play' by LUDI and presented in the list below, draw a clear portrait of the play and of the playing child.

- *The concept of frame.* Play is a special context in life, a frame that one can get in, get out, that can be suspended for a while, in which behaviours, meanings, rules and roles are different from reality. Players create, recognise and agree on this play frame, that is contemporarily invisible and concrete and that they inhabit and defend both from intruders and sceptics.

- *The need of doing.* Play is related to the human fundamental need to be active, to interact with the world around. The process of doing seems to be interesting per se, and more important than its results. Children themselves impose limitations and constraints to their activity, thus obtaining both the goals of being reassured by repetition and feeling challenged by novelty.

- *The role of imagination and fantasy.* Play is also the main door for entering 'another reality', for evoking situations, combining representations, developing thought; it is the door to the profusion of symbols, language, metaphors, creativity and imagination.

- *The importance of the rules.* Rules in play are not limited to games; they are rather intrinsic to all the kinds of play at any developmental age: first created by children themselves and later socially agreed-upon. According to Vygotskij, 'the essential attribute in play is a rule that has become a desire' and Bondioli underlines that children take pleasure in 'self-submitting to the rule of giving up spontaneous and impulsive actions'. In some cases, rules can put the players into trouble: getting out of it is the gist of play.

- *The social aspects of play.* Play is social in two main senses: because children learn to play in dual relationships or in groups, and because most of the types and modes of play require social contexts. Play relationships with peers are irreplaceable in childhood to learn by imitation, to face different opinions, to acknowledge the need for mediation, to develop skills of cooperation, to overcome conflicts. Adult and parental influence is vital for the child to start and learn how to play: at the beginning, they can be protagonist models, and then – by gradually fading their interaction – they can become prompters, scaffolders, companions, spectators. Please refer to Chapter 5 for a discussion on the role of an adult supporting children's play.

- *The play development in childhood.* Play develops and changes along childhood; it becomes more complex, it changes its features and its focus, by addressing different tools and/or ways to interpret the reality and the human beings. Research identified different types of play and showed that a given type of play prevails in certain developmental phases, then it merges with others, and it may disappear but also re-emerge in different forms, in different times of life.

Types of play

What are then these types of play? Play development has been described along two main dimensions, the cognitive and the social, which has been interpreted contemporarily as a consequence and as a cause of their growing complexity in time. After deep analysis on the field literature, LUDI has adopted the following classification of types of play.

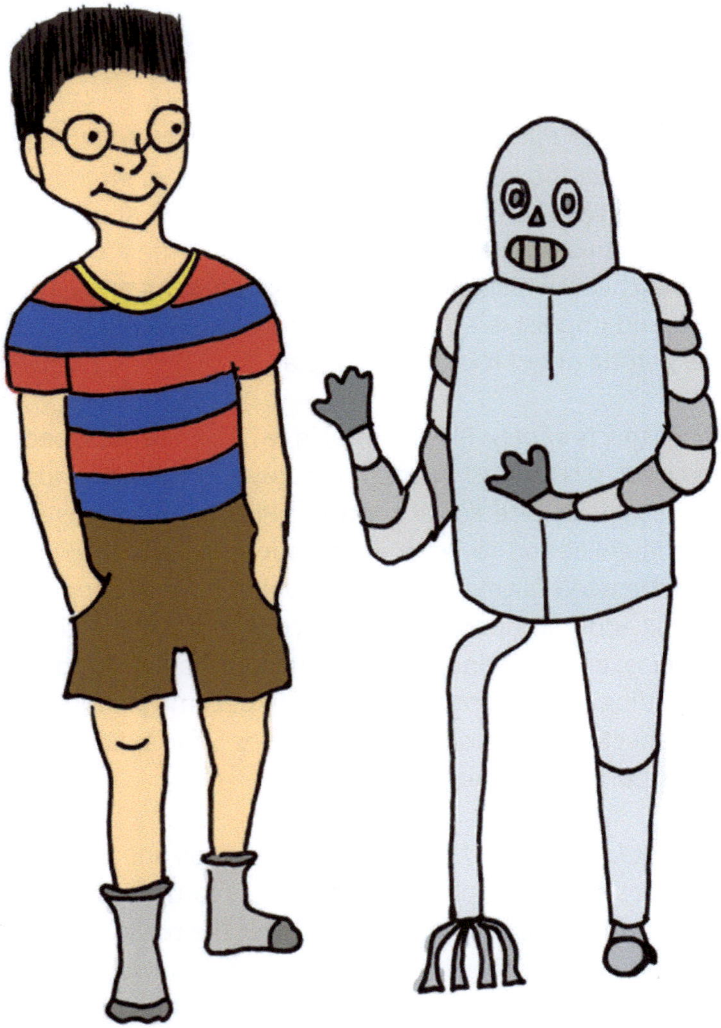

Jana, 16 years old, Croatia

Cognitive dimension

Practice play.

It is the first type of play that appears in life, related to body actions – from simple to complex – and to the visual and tactile experimentation of objects. Repetition is a typical characteristic of this type of play.

Symbolic play.

It starts around the second year of life, and it refers to the symbolic use of one's own body and of objects, as they were something else, to pretend and make-believe activities. The simplest form of this type of play is the simulation of action with the body – pretending to eat, to drive a car, etc.; the most complex is the role playing – acting roles and planning scenes for them.

Constructive play.

It consists in gathering, combining, arranging and fitting more elements to form a whole, and achieve a specific goal. The child combines abilities gained through practice and symbolic play, and the three types reciprocally co-exist and feed off each other.

Play with rules.

It includes play and games based on a specific code and rules accepted and followed by the players. It starts with simple rules invented by the players to make their play activities more challenging and it may evolve in the use of board games, as well as in sport activities.

Social dimension
Solitary play. The child plays alone and independently even if surrounded by others.
Parallel play. The child plays independently performing the same activity, at the same time, and in the same place of other persons, also engaged in play, without joining them.
Associative play. The child is focused on a separate activity with respect to his/her peers, but there is a considerable amount of sharing, lending, taking turns with them.
Cooperative play. Joining others in sustained engagement in activities with objects, toys, materials or games with a shared goal or purpose. Children can organize their play cooperatively with a common goal and are able to differentiate and assign roles.

Each type of play appears at a certain point of the child's life, usually according to the order shown in the table, in the form of an embryonic new group of behaviours, and it becomes more and more complex during time. Furthermore, soon each type of play intertwines with the other ones, which already belong to the child's repertoire, provoking changes in them; vice-versa, in some cases, very basic patterns of primitive types of play appear again to support more advanced play activities.

Play for the sake of play and play-like activities

In the history of education, play has not rarely been seen as useless, potentially distracting and subversive, unpredictable and uncontrollable; it was often repressed or at best channelled since it was deemed contrary to the seriousness of didactic engagement and schoolwork. Today, the commitment to play can be found in early childhood school programs in many different countries: dedicated spaces are organized, with appropriate materials and right time in the curriculum; nevertheless, even if play is accepted, in many cases it is still seen as a necessary outburst, sometimes relegated to the recess, where teachers and educators can ignore it.

Distinguished pedagogists and educators, however, realised that the strong potential of play to capture and maintain the child's attention on activities usually considered boring or difficult could be important for changing the climate of classrooms and family contexts and for making educational activities become closer to the child's propensities.

This is why the methodology of applying playfulness to the educational areas addressed to childhood was born; materials and tools were developed, working methodologies and strategies have spread that make learning more light, engaging, full of surprises and joy. Since then, children's play has become a useful stratagem for proposing learning activities, in schools, in other educational settings, at home. Playful activities are also presented, in the case of children with disabilities, in rehabilitation contexts. Many toy companies assure educational value on their products' packaging; schoolbooks are geared to the so-called gamification and are often accompanied by playful drill-and-practice software environments. However, the play adopted in these cases loses some peculiar features: for example, freedom, pure ludic spirit, transgression of rules, imagination and fantasy, autonomous initiative and choice. According to Visalberghi these activities, despite being amusing and fun, do not end in themselves, rather are 'controlled' by the adult and dominated by the educational final scope. He called them 'play-like activities'. Despite their importance, play-like activities do not cover all the forms play may assume, because they have pre-ordained educational goals.

It was the advent of the constructivist and active approaches in pedagogy and in psychology, about the second half of the last century, that brought a refreshing new tone in the childhood studies: children started to be considered the resilient protagonists of their own developmental process - they have rights, they are active constructors of knowledge, they are social beings and, thanks to their curiosity and their inexhaustible desire to solve the problems they face, they may be viewed also as researchers. According to the famous 'Reggio Emilia approach', as Hewett and some other authors recognize, every child should be given the opportunity to show which types of play attract him/her the most and to try further ones, so that new interests and evolving skills may be discovered and developed. Through play, the child will show desires and propensities, and will implement the best solutions to overcome the possible difficulties he/she may meet.

Play as such, play for the sake of play, responds only to the play needs and wishes of the child; it develops and stops for its own reasons, it does not have constraints that are not decided by the child him or herself. Play for the sake of play contains the exact 'rate' and type of fun and challenge that the child wants. It favours experimentation, exploration, curiosity, imagination because it is intrinsically driven; due to its inherent flexibility, it can stop at any time and re-start all of a sudden, it tolerates changing rules under the only obligation of an agreement among players. It is totally adherent to the child's personal idea of what is compelling, pleasant and exciting for him/her, because it is the child who continuously invents and monitors it. It makes it possible to create fantastic worlds only inhabited by the child with his or her imaginary playmates.

Why is play important?

But if fun produced by play is a formidable spring to involve the child in activities that are considered important by the adults, what about play for the sake of play? If this one is just recreation and leisure, why should it be considered so important?

The main reason is that it is through play that children develop and grow up as human beings: persons able to purposefully act on their life environments and to positively take part into society.

Freedom, curiosity, imagination, adherence to – and subversion of – rules, concentration, repetition, satisfaction, set up of goals, planning, problem solving are only some of the traits that are put into action while playing. The quality and the range of different play experiences made by a child will pave the way to an adult rich in resources, creativity, self-confidence, sociability and cheerfulness; the complete and absolute happiness provoked by play will remain one of the most powerful feelings experienced in life.

However, it is impossible to determine what children might learn when they play for the sole sake of play: it will depend on the chosen type of play, on the way the play activity is concretely put into action, on the companions' quality of participation, on the contexts where play happens. They might learn psychomotor and cognitive abilities – how to be effective in throwing a ball, to climb a tree, to solve an impasse in a board game, to build a rudimentary canoe by oneself, to use irony, metaphors and fantasy in general, to plan a strategy, etc.; social abilities – how to involve peers in a game, to coordinate the roles, to mediate during conflicts, to argue one's reasons, to keep secrets, to conceal a feeling or an idea, etc.; emotional abilities – how to recognize one's own limits, to accept defeat, to perceive and enjoy happiness or to cope with fear and with exhaustion.

Above all, they will learn a lot about themselves – their preferences, abilities, inclinations – and about the others – how to recognize their intentions and feelings, how to relate with them, how different or unpredictable their emotions and behaviours may be. They may develop self-confidence on their own strengths and may use the privileged and protected situation of play to learn how to overcome their weaknesses.

Play for the sake of play is also important for the large amount of information the observer might gather from it on the individual child's ability, cognitive styles, overall well-being and sociability.

A parent, an educator or a practitioner can enter the child's play to improve, increase, and develop it; not for reaching external goals, not to turn it into a play-like activity, but only to pursue objectives inherent to the play itself. Learning to enter children's play, with full awareness of one's own adulthood, but maintaining and respecting the constraints and limitations of the play that children are actually playing and adopting the appropriate scaffolding strategies to support the interactions between children and between the child and the adult, is a new competence for adults to reach: becoming able to work behind the scenes, preparing the play materials and contexts and assuring the right climate for the carrying out of the play activity. Guidelines to achieve this are provided in Chapter 5.

Conclusion

Even if we do not know why play exists or even if putting this question has any reasonable sense, for sure play is an irreplaceable apprenticeship for life and a continuous source of serenity.

In spite of being studied for centuries, play still preserves a fascinating air of mystery, for its peculiar characteristics that make it unmistakable and powerful.

Dozens of definitions and descriptions of play have been proposed in the related fields of study. In this chapter, the definition of play adopted by LUDI has been discussed, and some important traits have been described, together with a consistent classification of the types of play. To understand and interpret in-depth the child's play, in fact, a clear framework is needed. When a child plays freely, without any limitation, he/she does a very special activity and always choses a specific type of play, or a mix of types. Referring to this activity simply as 'free play' is not exhaustive enough; we should instead be aware of what concept of play we are using, and which type of play is involved: because each type of play has its own characteristics, constraints and development possibilities.

This is particularly true in the case of play for the sake of play, intrinsically motivated and autonomously initiated, that we mostly want to pursue for children with disabilities.

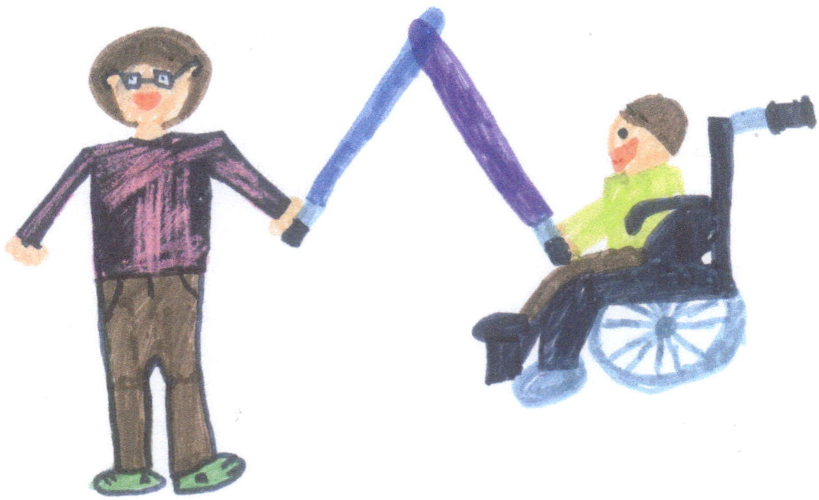

Rita, 9 years old, Spain

2

Do children with disabilities play?

Serenella Besio and Vaska Stancheva-Popkostadinova

In the previous chapter, we have defined what is play for the sake of play and described its importance for every child's harmonious development and well-being. Does it also apply for children with disabilities? And are children with disabilities interested in play and capable of playing? Before answering thes questions, let us start by defining the concept of disability.

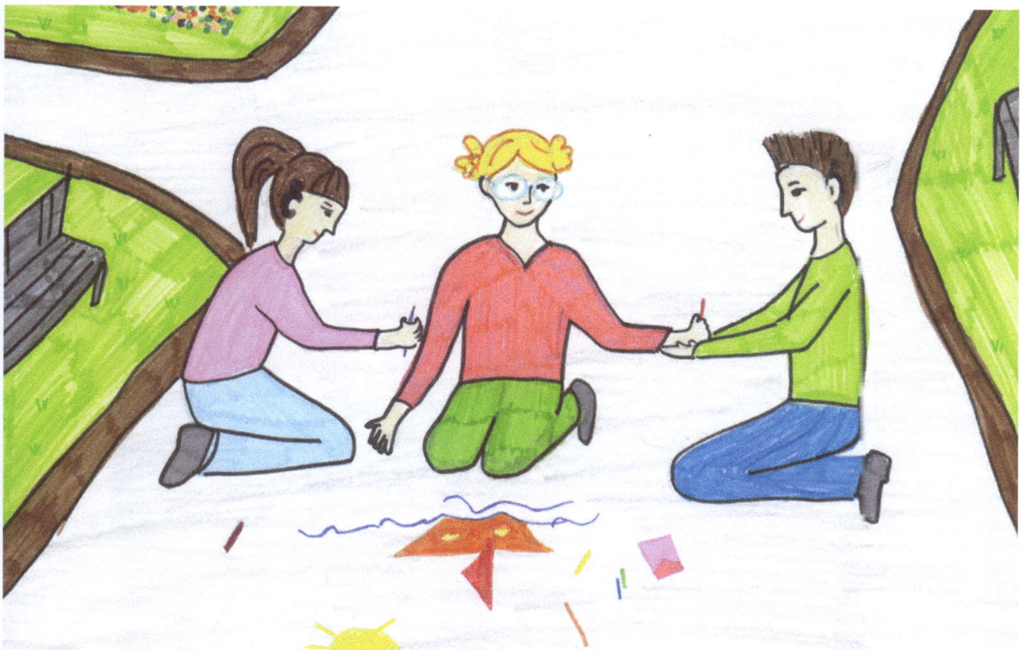

Darina, 12 years old, Bulgaria

What is disability?

In 2001, the World Health Organisation (WHO) adopted the bio-psycho--social model to describe human functioning and the conditions of health and disability, by launching the International Classification of Functioning, Disability and Health (ICF). ICF represents the result of a scientific and socio-political debate about the definition of disability and the health model that underlies it. Prior to this, two models have existed: first the bio-medical, which attributed to the body impairment the main responsibility for disability and social disadvantage; then the social model, which has strongly emphasised the role played by physical barriers and social attitudes in producing the restrictions to participation faced by persons with disabilities. In the first case, solutions should be found and planned within the health system, in rehabilitation and intervention – ultimately within a perspective of separation and specialisation; in the second case, the solutions must be identified at the level of social and political programming, as well as in the change of collective attitudes – everyone's participation in community life and its opportunities must be guaranteed.

The bio-psycho-social model accepted to some extent the fundamental statements of the two previous ones and seeks, on the one hand, to balance the various elements that can favour or determine a condition of disability and, on the other, to highlight the numerous and constant interactions between them. The following figure represents the main concept of ICF.

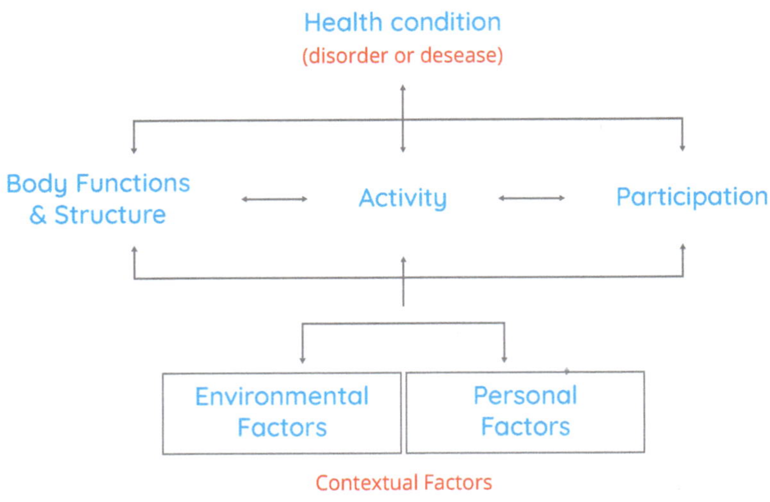

Interactions between the components of the WHO ICF model

Within the ICF framework, functioning or disability are closely connected to biological factors, environmental factors and personal factors, each of them bringing a positive or negative contribution to the two main components of the individuals' life, which are the activity and the participation. Disability is defined as 'an umbrella term for impairment, activity limitation and participation restriction. It denotes the negative aspects of the interactions between an individual (with a health condition) and the individual's contextual factors (environmental and personal factors)'. More precisely, ICF asserts that 'disability is characterised as the outcome or the result of a complex relationship between an individual's health condition and personal factors, and of the external factors that represent the circumstances in which the individual lives. Because of this relationship, different environments may have a very different impact on the same individual with a given health condition. An environment with barriers, or without facilitators, will restrict the individual performance; other environments that are more facilitating, may increase the performance. Society may hinder an individual's performance because either it creates barriers (e.g. inaccessible buildings) or it does not provide facilitators (e.g. unavailability of assistive devices)'.

The purpose of the ICF is not to classify individuals, rather to put into evidence the complex relations between possible impairments of body functions or structures and the individual's activity limitations or participation restrictions, on the one hand, and the influence of the environmental factors as barriers or facilitators, on the other hand. Accordingly, ICF focuses on the description of functional characteristics, thus abandoning the stigmatizing approach to disability based on diseases, disorders or other health conditions.

The ICF establishes the Activity and the Participation as main components of the individuals' health, which can reveal and give information on functioning or disability. In order to take part in activities and to participate in life, people need both to have the required capacity and to be able to perform within a given environment. While within the model capacity is defined as the highest level of a person's functioning in a 'standardised environment', performance is defined as what the person is in fact able to do in his/her usual environments of life. It is exactly thanks to this distinction that ICF paves the way to understanding the determinant role of environmental factors in influencing the functioning of an individual. These factors may intervene in favour of the individual's performance, thus being considered facilitators, when thanks to them the individual's performance improves with respect to what is expected from the capacity analysis. On the contrary, they are considered as barriers, when their presence hinders or prevents the individual from exploiting his/her full capacity and/or performance.

The WHO framework has the strength and the value of a philosophical Manifesto on human beings and their societies: men and women are considered active since their birth and throughout their life, because one of their innate instincts is the action on the world around them, and are intended as fully participating into this world – with nature, with other humans, with artefacts. Activity is essential for the individual's development and life, and it may happen only within the environments in which he/she lives, and thanks to social participation: on this point ICF converges with the ecological views of development as a fruitful and mutual encounter between the person and the environment. Which different approach could better admit and explain the children's play?

Play and children with disabilities

Children's most important activity is play. Through play, as already mentioned, they learn, they experiment, they grow, they become social companions and they explore and interact with their life contexts.

Play has been expressly included in the 'International Classification of Functioning, Disability and Health: Children & Youth Version' (ICF-CY), the version of ICF devoted to children and their specificities, published in 2006. In this way, WHO recognises that play is a substantial component of the child's health, playing a central role in the child's life not only as an activity, but also as a crucial occasion to meet the others, to interact with them and to take part in his/her contexts of life. As a consequence, any action aiming at safeguarding and implementing a good children's health status should address play and do it from the biological, the psychological, and the social and environmental perspectives.

Play, in fact, represents a peculiar opportunity for building social inclusion. The contexts in which children's play occurs are an ideal and fertile soil for social development, to nurture and support the adoption of attitudes of collaboration and mutual respectful interest, to educate to inter-individual differences and foster integration, allowing everyone to participate in the best way and to have the opportunity to choose. Within inclusive play contexts, all children may have the opportunity to share spaces, objects, intentions and rules, they can test their abilities, imitate the others or being models for them, or they can even refuse to play and communicate their 'getting out of the play'. They should have the opportunity to win, to lose, to collaborate, to build together, to negotiate and to argue, to be wrong, to explore, to feel happy, scared, excited, concentrated.

This is true for all children, regardless of possible impairments: all children can in fact play, if environmental and personal factors are able to accommodate children with disabilities' particular needs. And play is also a very special and irreplaceable life context to foster true inclusion for children with disabilities, since it provides opportunities to interacting with others, on the basis of fun and reciprocal acceptance.

Children who experience some types of impairment need and want to play. However, they may meet numerous obstacles, such as difficulties in initiating and carrying out play, making it more complex, understanding or applying some rules, sharing it with other peers; they may sometimes be scared by some aspects of the play contexts or tools, or be deprived of leisure time by their daily schedule, often full of rehabilitative activities. In some cases, an impaired child may seem stuck in a developmental phase without proceeding to explore new types of play, preferring to repeat those who is already accustomed to. In other cases, an impaired child expresses the interest in particular ludic activities that supposedly are not suited to him/her (e.g. playing ball for a blind child, running for a child with cerebral palsy). Some children may conceive only the real world and pretend or role play seems abstruse and even frightening to them; others would like to take part in group games but they feel (or are) excluded from peers and remain on the outskirts.

The most frequent occasions to play for children with disabilities are proposed to them by adults within dyadic relationships. However, for rehabilitation professionals, medical doctors and special educators – whom they meet almost every day – play is often a disguise for exercise and functional improvement. This habit is then transferred to home, because parents tend to reproduce, in the same playful way, those training activities which are well tested and do not challenge them. In addition, leisure time, where new play occasions and desires might arise, and play for the sake of play might occur, is reduced for these families due to many commitments. Please refer to Chapter 3 for a discussion on the barriers to play faced by children with disabilities.

The different types of play identified in Chapter 1 are experimented by children along their development, in relation to their preferences and dispositions, certainly influenced by the characteristics of their functioning. Nevertheless, the children's context has a determinant role: the presence of siblings, the lifestyle (e.g. open to the outdoor and natural environments or not, full of relationships or not), the adults' ideas on the importance of play, the ludic experience of parents, the quality of inclusive policies in their countries, etc. This chapter will briefly discuss the impact of health conditions, body functions and structures on play. Environmental and personal factors will then be discussed in the following chapters providing specific guidelines to support children with disabilities' play.

Types of disabilities and play

As discussed above, disability is a wrong or critical encounter between the physical, the psychological and the contextual characteristics. This paragraph is mainly devoted to consider more in-depth the impact of the different kinds of impairments on play.

The LUDI Classification of Disabilities, which is the result of an on-purpose study, is reported in the following Table.

LUDI categories of disabilities
Mental or intellectual disability (mild, moderate, severe, profound)
Hearing impairment (partial hearing impairment, deafness)
Visual impairment (partial visual impairment, blindness)
Communication disorder (language disorder)
Physical impairment (mild, moderate, severe)
Autism Spectrum Disorders
Multiple disabilities

For each of these categories of disability it is possible to describe the most frequent physical impairments and the related functional limitations. However, it is important to point out that, if this allows to pay particular attention to certain developmental areas that may be compromised, it is not intended in any way to standardise the children who have the same type of impairment, thus disregarding inter-individual differences.

On the contrary, it should be clear that every child is different from the other ones, due to personal factors (such as the family, its educational style, the geographical area in which they live, with its characteristics and traditions, the gender, personality traits, preferences, etc.) as well as to the individual biogenetic heritage.

Mental and intellectual disabilities

Children with mental and intellectual disabilities may show an overall delayed development and a very particular functioning of mental skills; every acquisition needs a long period of consolidation, through frequent repetitions and recalls. They also meet difficulties in understanding what happens around them, in relating events to their possible causes and also in decoding and acquiring the verbal language. They may need support in learning from experience, often due to memory problems and to a kind of reluctance towards environmental exploration. Social relationships may be challenging too, in some cases they prefer solitary and isolate activities, in other they may behave in a too intrusive way. All these functional aspects may delay and affect both practice and pretend or symbolic play.

Mental or intellectual disabilities imply – to various degrees – deficits in reasoning, problem solving, abstract thinking, judgement, as well as deficits in adaptive functioning, including social and practical difficulties; they may also influence a refined and effective movement coordination. These functional aspects may affect constructive play and rule-based play.

As youngsters, they hardly succeed in developing an adequate self-consciousness; the frequent lack of awareness about their difficulties may be a critical aspect that educators should carefully consider when establishing inclusive play contexts and activities.

Hearing impairments

A hearing loss may prevent a child from totally or partially perceiving sounds. This has, of course, important consequences on the child's development, mainly related to his/her participation to the environmental events, if the information is prevailingly conveyed by sounds, especially in the case of verbal language.

While practice and constructive play are not influenced that much by this kind of impairment (except when the activity or the toy are mainly based on sounds), symbolic play may be hugely affected, since it makes a large use of communication and verbal exchanges and it is mainly held in group. The case of games is even more complicated: in fact, the rules might represent a bias, if they are not clearly explained and understood.

The knowledge and use of Sign Language from the very early childhood may help a lot, especially if this competence is shared among a group of peers, regardless of whether they are hearing children or not.

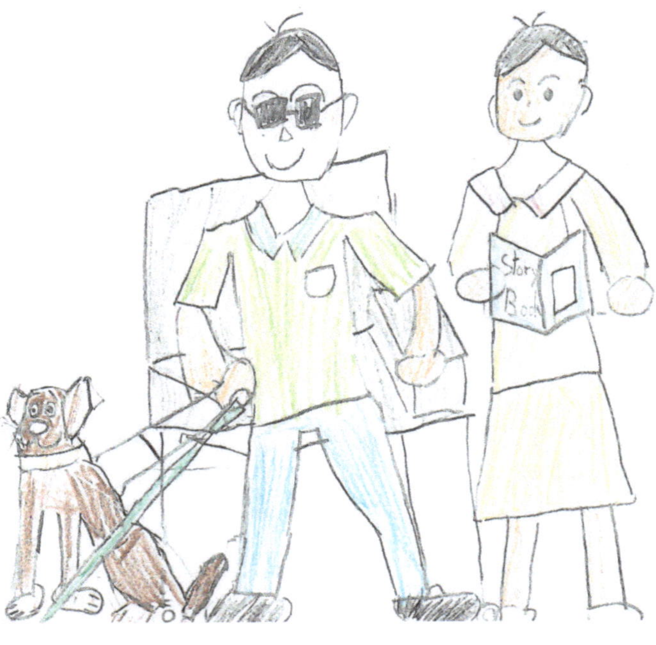

Roberto, 8 years old, Malta

Visual impairments

A functional limitation of the vision system that cannot be compensated by usual aids may provoke a large range of visual loss, from low vision to blindness. Children with visual impairment may experience many difficulties in relating to the environments and the objects around them; they must rely mainly on hearing and touch to explore the space and to act within it, but this implies longer times (with respect to their peers) in understanding what things are made of, how they work, what happens and what they can expect from the situations and the persons around. For these reasons, they may find it difficult to develop any type of play.

Practice and constructive play may be delayed or deprived because they require children with visual impairments to relate with the built world. Quite paradoxically, pretend play may be tricky because their way to interpret the world is necessarily strictly based on fixed rules – and thus it is difficult for them to interpret one object 'as if it was' another one, similar but not the same.

On the other hand, they may prove very skilled in symbolic play activities based on verbal language (e.g. fantasy tales, theatre representations, etc.) as well as in rule-based games, if the tools used are accessible to them. Generally speaking, in fact, their cognitive and language abilities are preserved and sometimes they become their prevailing and brilliant interaction channel with the others.

Acquiring a satisfying and rich social competence often proves difficult for visually impaired children, especially with sighted peers; this contributes to provoke their predominant disposition towards solitary play or in small groups. However, collaborative play and in bigger inclusive groups may be pursued and obtained: some experiences of adapted and inclusive sport activities are a very effective demonstration of possible future exploitations.

Communication disorders

Deficits in language and speech are considered as a specific area of impairments, because they may be experienced without connections to other disabilities.

These disorders may affect social participation and occupational performance; preschool children linger long in the stage of practice play with respect to their peers, while symbolic play is mastered by them more slowly and in a less creative way. Symbolic play may be hindered by the difficulty to agree with the others about pretending an object is something else, or in building up play situations with roles, conversations, etc. They tend to play with toys in a solitary and silent way; furthermore, their language may be considered ineffective or not clear enough by their peers, thus diminishing their active participation to social play activities.

When they become older, their communication impairments may create difficulties in handling peer conflict and in behaving in an assertive way: all the play activities in which negotiation, mediation, explaining one's own points of view are necessary can be challenging for children with communication disorders. This has important consequences, on the one hand, on their development of skills needed for rule-based games and, on the other hand, on their participation to social play in general.

Physical impairments

Physical impairments, that may be acquired or congenital, affect at various degrees the physical ability to move, to coordinate actions, to perform physical and motor daily life tasks independently. The great variety of causes of physical impairments may create very different types of limitations to functioning; in some cases, the physical impairment is associated with other types of disabilities – sensory, intellectual, neuropsychological – and this, of course, creates different life situations.

Generally speaking, children with physical impairments experience difficulty in concretely interacting with the environment around them, using objects and toys. Exploring and moving in the space may prove very difficult for them and even impossible without any support. Naturally, this prevents or makes it very challenging the practice and the constructive types of play. According to some studies - but this is a vital issue of discussion now in research – this deprivation of a concrete experimentation with the built reality may in turn have other detrimental effects in reasoning, representation and abstraction skills development.

The participation of children with physical impairment to symbolic play might be greatly compromised by their motor impairments, but – moreover when the cognitive abilities are safeguarded – it can also be strongly supported by imagination and fantasy, and concretely accomplished thanks to the use of virtual environments and technical aids. They may also play rule-based games with their peers on a digital support if available. A possible issue in this case may be the response speed required by the game, because children's movements might be slower than expected or required, and regulation measures should be identified accordingly.

Very often, children with physical impairments need the adoption of various assistive devices and support and this implies a special organisation of their daily life and of the spaces where they live; this may create risks of participation restrictions. In order to avoid it, inclusive play plans should then take into careful consideration the practical, technical and logistical aspects of the activities.

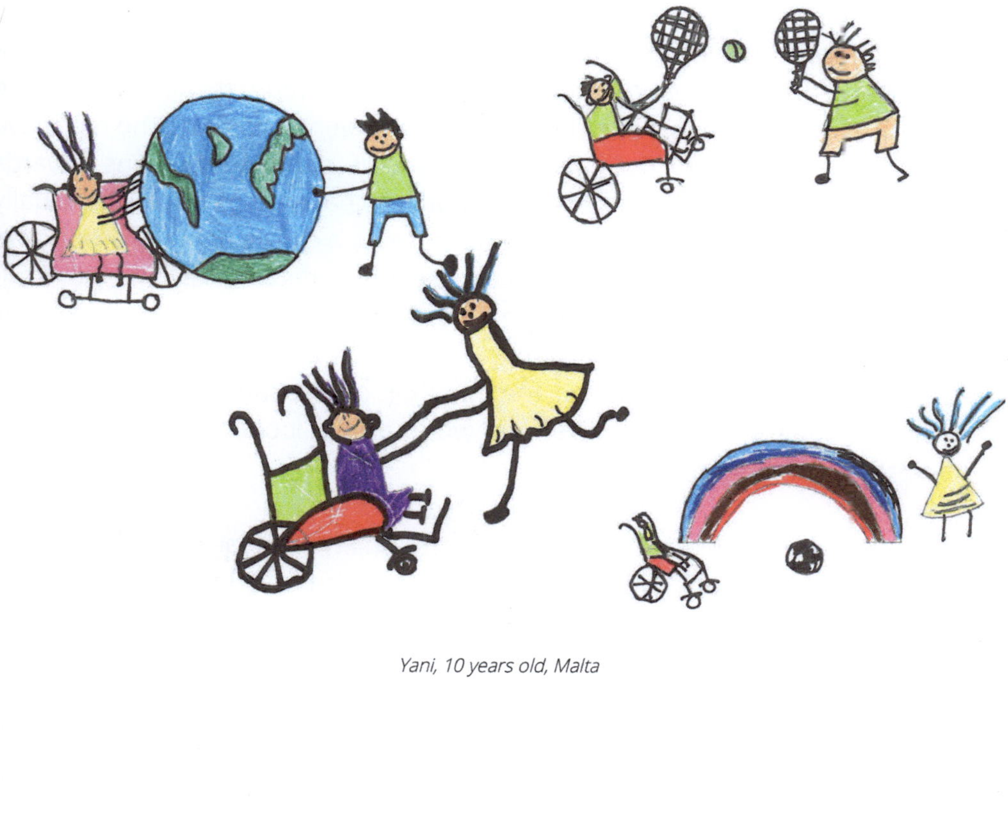

Yani, 10 years old, Malta

Autism spectrum disorders

Children with Autism Spectrum Disorders (ASD) show restrictive, repetitive patterns of behaviour and experience also deficits in social communication and social interaction. This group of disorders is described as a 'spectrum', to underline that various areas and degrees of limitations may be involved and that, as a consequence, the range of possible manifestations is really wide and differs from one individual to another.

Nevertheless, the play skills of children with ASD may be severely influenced by the central role of their impairments in the social and the communication areas; in addition, it should be reminded that an intellectual disability is often associated with these disorders, together with sensory dysfunctions (that may take the form of over-sensitivity as well as insensitivity to stimuli), delayed or reduced verbal communication, difficulties in emotional development.

Children with ASD are usually described as less interested in play activities than their typically developing peers. Their difficulties in the gross and fine psychomotor and coordination areas may be related to their little interest into the objects and how they work, which decreases the rate and the quality of the practice type of play, even if this observation seems contradicted as soon as they concentrate on a detail of an object or a particular use of it. However, in this case the repetitive behaviours they adopt are not perceived as playful, rather as a means towards social isolation. Constructive play may be equally challenging, since it is usually based on the application of fine motor skills to create a consistent final product. In fact, while they have the great ability to concentrate on details, they find it difficult to foresee an overall form, built by assembling small pieces. Pretend and symbolic play – as studies in the field widely confirm – are affected by their social difficulties, for example in sharing with another the attention on the same activity or object, or in understanding the perspective from which a peer looks at (or evaluates, or perceives) the same event.

Pretend and symbolic play require the ability to deal with fantasy and imagination, to look to possible worlds and the possible life within them, and these abilities are not easy to achieve by children with ASD.

The difficulty to adopt the other's perspective is also what mainly impedes children with autism spectrum disorders to show an autonomous interest into rule-based play, and to take part in it. It may also justify why collaborative and social play with peers is less frequent with them. Nevertheless, it is not rare to observe that, once a child with ASD finds a play companion interested in the same specialised activities he/she wishes and is able to do, the child shows great pleasure in sharing them.

Multiple disabilities

Today there is not a consensus on a unique definition of multiple disability. What is anyway clear is that this expression is related to multiple severe impairments experienced by the same individual, which creates severe conditions that need to be accommodated by very specialised programs. Children with multiple disabilities have huge problems in receiving and decoding information coming from the environment, and they often live in a condition of misinformation that hugely interferes with their play skills. They may show unexpected responses to the proposed ludic activities, may require a lot of time in processing the stimuli, or exhibit intense reactions. Social skills are usually severely compromised, and they often tend to isolation and to use the objects for self-stimulation or stereotypical behaviours. Involvement in pretend and symbolic play, and even more in rule-based play, is usually hard to achieve. Cooperative and social play is also challenging.

In this case, researchers have mainly concentrated their studies on play as one of the prevailing means to support the development of possible new skills by children with multiple disabilities: improving perception, movement, communication and socialisation have been the goals established in these works. The right space setting and equipment availability are of utmost importance for supporting their play.

Conclusion

Do children with disabilities play? Yes, they do and they can. And they could play more, and better, if the most suitable and accurate solutions to overcome limitations and restrictions to play are found, created or invented.

To reach this objective, to make play possible, playful, fully satisfactory, autonomous and inclusive at the same time, the three components of the ICF – body functions and structures, activity and participation, and environment – should be considered altogether.

Turning the spotlight on infant play thus, means considering various aspects of the child's life and environment, including his/her body, without putting them in a hierarchy but rather studying their interdependencies: a complex task that requires competence, specialised observation ability, intuitive capability and the availability of a lot of information.

In this chapter, a first step towards the design of this interdependency has been undertaken, since the main functional characteristics of the different categories of disabilities singled out by LUDI have been presented, in relation to the types of play identified. Even if they should be considered in the light of the high variability existing between individuals, this presentation aims to contribute to build up an overall and multidisciplinary knowledge on play and children with disabilities.

In the next chapters, the environmental factors will be treated in-depth so that, at the end, it will become clear that, under proper conditions, children with disabilities can enjoy the ludic experience in all its richness, engaging in fun, satisfying and challenging play activities.

3

What barriers to play do children with disabilities face?

Helen Lynch and Alice Moore

When your child has a disability, his or her play opportunities may be impacted: their play may be experienced as more limiting. In fact, research shows that children with disabilities can experience more restrictions, fewer opportunities, less access, and less range of ability for play compared to other children. In recent research, this has been attributed to significant problems in the environment: the PHYSICAL, SOCIO-CULTURAL, and POLITICAL environment. Many people view this as an interdependent issue: we cannot look at one aspect alone but need to address this problem from each perspective. Most importantly, we need to start with the child, and the rights of the child to play.

This chapter begins with presenting an overview of play in relation to the rights of the child. First, the context is set by examining the concept of children as rights holders, and the importance of play as a right for all children through an overview of the United Nations Convention on the Rights of the Child (UNCRC). Barriers to play will then be outlined in contrast to this, and an overview will be presented of some more recent developments in relation to making progress on implementing the child's right to play for all children.

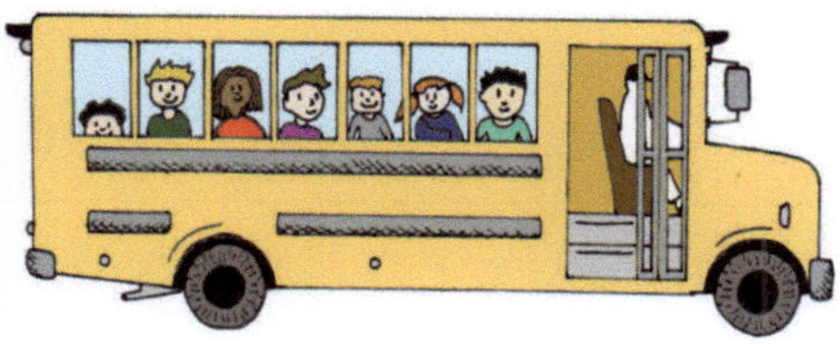

Lara, 16 years old, Croatia

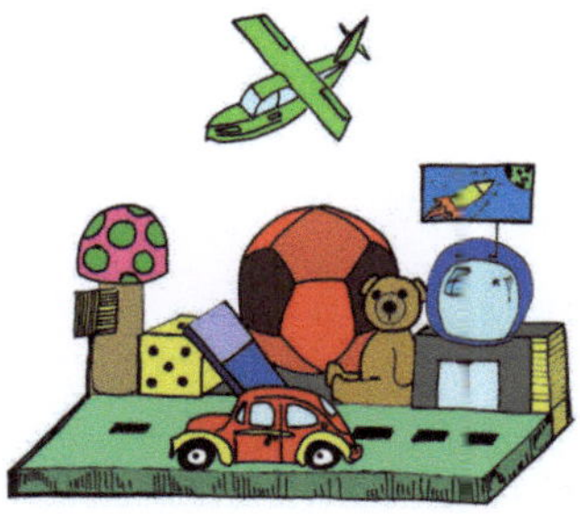

Miljan, 16 years old, Croatia

Key policies

1. United Nations Convention on the Rights of the Child (UNCRC), 1989
2. United Nations Convention on the Rights of Persons with Disabilities (UNCRPD), 2007
3. General Comments No. 9, 2006 and No. 17, 2013
4. International Play Association Play for Children with Disabilities, 2015
5. LUDI Position Statement on Play and the Rights of Children with Disabilities, 2017

Is play a right? The UNCRC

When the United Nations Convention on the Rights of the Child was first published, it represented an international recognition and commitment to protecting and promoting children's rights to lead rich and fulfilled lives. The UNCRC was published in 1989 and was written for all children across the world. It consists of 54 articles, targeting human, social and economic rights, frequently grouped into three main areas: the three P's of Protection, Participation, and Provision. Of most relevance to this chapter is Article 31: the right to play.

Article 31 of the UNCRC

That every child has the right to rest and leisure, to engage in play and recreational activities appropriate to the age of the child and to participate freely in cultural life and the arts. That member governments shall respect and promote the right of the child to participate fully in cultural and artistic life and shall encourage the provision of appropriate and equal opportunities for cultural, artistic, recreational and leisure activity.

The right to play and leisure was included in the UNCRC because of the fundamental place that play holds in relation to childhood: play is central to how a child participates in the world; it underpins healthy development, well-being, quality of life, socio-cultural participation, resilience, and creativity. This in turn means that the right to play is **interdependent** on the right to health and the right to education: a rights-based approach to health, education or social inclusion therefore needs to include the right to play.

In the UNCRC, there are four other articles that are often called cross-cutting or general principles:

- Article 2 on non-discrimination;
- Article 3 on best interests of the child;
- Article 6 on right to life, survival, and development;
- Article 12 on right to be heard.

Each of these four principles are relevant to ensuring the right conditions for play are provided for every child, and particularly for children with disabilities.

A fundamental issue that is at the foundation of the convention is that of children as rights-holders. Although all member states of the United Nations (UN) have signed the UNCRC, the implementation differs in respect of this issue. For example, in a review of the UNCRC and its implementation, researchers found that analysing the perspective of children as rights-holders was a crucial aspect: countries (such as Belgium, Norway and Spain) who had incorporated the UNCRC had a culture of respect for children's rights and viewed children as rights-holders. This reflects the changing nature of society in many developed countries: children are viewed as having a voice, and of being experts on their own lives. This position has led to a whole movement across Europe to promote children's participation (an implementation of Article 12, UNCRC). For example, in 2016 the Council of Europe published a toolkit to examine children's participation in Europe, while in Ireland the government established a participation hub to progress this agenda for children's rights nationally.

Case Study example: Impact of the UNCRC - Development of a National Policy for Play, Ireland

Ireland became one of the first countries in Europe to produce a detailed national policy on play. In March 2004, the Government of Ireland produced 'Ready, Steady, Play! A National Play Policy' to honour commitments made in the UNCRC, which Ireland ratified in 1992. The policy illustrated the Government's recognition of the importance of play, and a commitment to making sure that equitable and inclusive play is facilitated for all children, particularly children who are marginalised, disadvantaged or who have a disability. The policy was implemented in Ireland in 2004 and is currently being reviewed.

What happened since 1989

Since 1989, the international community of States (countries) adopted this UNCRC convention formally so that now (in 2018) almost all United Nations member states have ratified it. In a UNICEF review (2012) of the implementation of the UNCRC, examples of good practice were presented that included the use of non-legal measures such as the development of national strategies for children and establishing detailed data sets on children's lives. However, the majority of countries had not developed legal measures that would give more robust commitment to implementation. This report acknowledged the challenges of implementing the UNCRC and the wide variety of different approaches across European countries in doing so. Although the review did not target play rights specifically, it highlights the difficulties in implementing international policy at national context.

Therefore, it is important to explore and understand the barriers that exist to providing for play, in order to consider what we can do to progress the play agenda for children with disabilities and ensure their rights to play are taken seriously.

Barriers to play: lack of political commitment to implementing the right to play

The political environment is closely linked to the economic environment, as national funding typically follows legislation and policies to support government initiatives.

- Despite the ratification of the UNCRC across Europe and beyond, to date, few countries have developed national plans in relation to play, and few have guidelines on providing play for all children including those with disabilities. In an online survey of 16 European countries in 2017, it was found that play policies had been developed only in two countries: in Ireland and in the UK (in the four regions: Northern Ireland, Wales, Scotland, and England).

- In a scoping review of evidence on usability and accessibility of playgrounds, researchers found that few national guidelines exist to inform design of inclusive playgrounds. This leads to national provision of playgrounds that are not designed for children of varied abilities, resulting in exclusion and inequality.

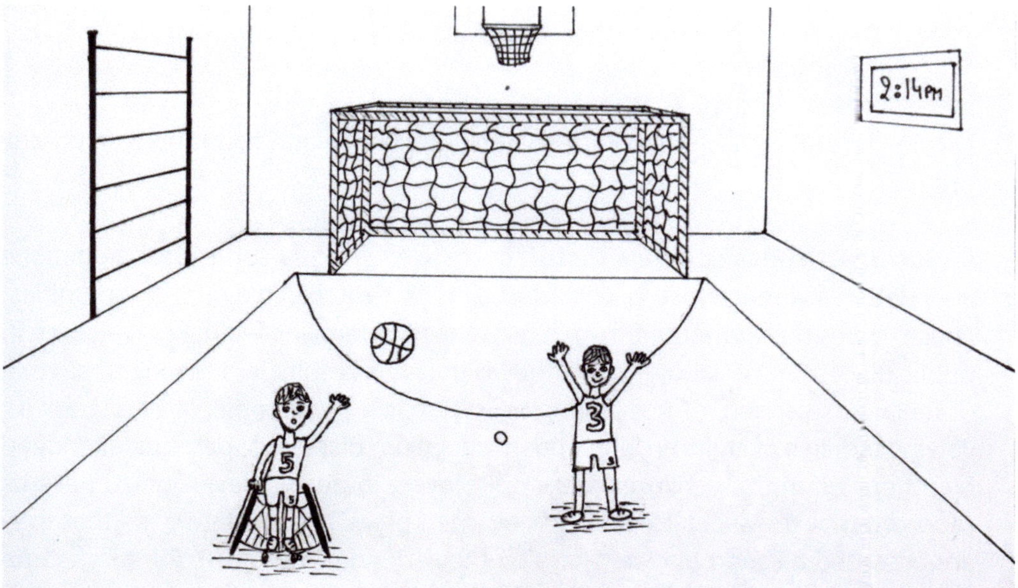

Myrthe, 15 years old, the Netherlands

- In a study in Sweden with municipal play providers, researchers found that there was a significant lack of knowledge about the play needs of children with disabilities, when designing or planning for developing playspaces in local communities.

- Although few studies have analysed why these problems arise in implementing the UNCRC, one study has reported some data to throw some light onto the issue. In a review of the implementation of Article 31 in the UK, researchers found that there was a lack of a rights-based perspective in implementation strategies being adopted, and argued that greater leadership was needed from the UN Committee on the Rights of the Child, such as to provide robust monitoring. Problems identified included the overly broad terms of the article leaving states unclear as to how to interpret play and play needs adequately.

Overall, it seems that when play is not taken seriously in national policy, play is poorly funded locally. This is an example of how the political, socio-cultural, and physical environments are closely interdependent.

Barriers to play: different values and attitudes in the socio-cultural environment

The socio-cultural environment for play includes family and community contexts, among others.

- **Social attitudes can be a factor:** there are currently some strong opinions and debates about what is considered as 'acceptable play' in communities. These issues have emerged from experiences of families feeling unwelcome in public places. Some studies have shown that this results in a feeling of stigma, of feeling ostracised, of not belonging in public. For example, in one study involving families of children with autism spectrum disorders, parents felt judged by others when their children were out playing in public playgrounds. Parents reported that they seek to ensure their child plays 'appropriately', so that they are accepted as good play partners by their friends. Therefore, for some families, the issue of what play is acceptable or appropriate is a big issue.

- Other socio-cultural studies with parents have identified that parents struggle with managing the child's identity in varied social settings due to social attitudes, where disability is viewed as a tragedy.

- **Health and education contexts** where play is not valued: it is a sad reflection of our societies if we forget about the importance of play. As a therapist, I regret the times I did not remember to build in authentic play goals together with the families I used to work with. 'Authentic play goals' refers to the fact that in many cases, therapists actually use play to build skills, e.g. to teach the child fine-motor skills or to improve manipulation. In a study of therapists in Ireland, Sweden, and Switzerland, for example, researchers found that the majority used play in this way. Few therapists thought of enabling play in families as an aim for its own value: for fun, for well-being, for family relationships. Family life is sustained when family members can develop and enjoy activities such as play together.

- **Family values and attitudes** are also a contributing factor: for example, when a child has a disability, many families are challenged to provide significant time to practice skills, follow up on education, rehabilitation or therapy schedules, and time is limited for play. It may be that parents feel guilty about not working with the child when they have time, yet all families need playtime.

Among play researchers in recent years, there is a growing realisation that there is a lack of knowledge about play for the sake of play, among many adults who care for children. Therefore, enabling play for children with disabilities is a complex issue, which warrants attention to knowledge, awareness, attitudes, and beliefs.

Barriers to play: physical environment

While significant barriers in the social and political environment have been presented, there are equally significant barriers in the physical environment to consider. Indeed, some studies have shown that if barriers in the physical environment are tackled, then social barriers can be more easily addressed.

- Studies have identified that the lack of physical access is a main barrier to participation of children with disabilities in community activities in many countries. Physical access refers to many design issues such as having pathways, entrances, and facilities designed for children of all abilities, so that a child who uses a wheelchair, for example, can access the swimming pool or enter the playground and use the equipment there. In one study of 57 playgrounds in the USA, researchers found that only 5% of routes and pathways met the standards set out by legislation for accessibility.

- Few studies have explored the physical environmental needs of children with other needs such as sensory or cognitive impairments. Therefore, a further barrier exists in relation to our lack of data on children with different needs.

- Where no or few guidelines exist for guiding local authorities on how best to provide for inclusive playspaces, many children with disabilities are excluded from playing with their friends. In a number of studies in Sweden, researchers found that children of varied abilities valued playgrounds as a place for play, but did not find playgrounds to be inclusive, or equitable places for play.

- Although the UNCRC establishes the need for children to be involved in matters that affect them such as in developing playspaces, no research has been published to date on children with disability and their engagement in designing for play.

So, with these barriers in mind, what else has been developed internationally in relation to addressing the rights to play for children with disability? The next section presents a brief introduction to key documents that guide us into the next phase of enabling play as an issue of rights.

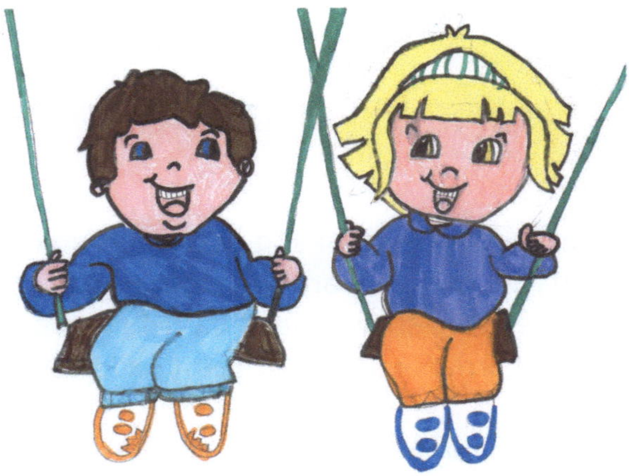

Eduardo, 7 years old, Italy

Strengthening the policy context: Play for Children with Disabilities - General Comment No. 9, 2006

When the UN adopts conventions and when states ratify them, there follows phases of implementation and review. Consequently, the UN works on what are called General Comments, to help strengthen the understanding of articles to support the interpretation of provisions within each convention. For example, since the UNCRC was ratified, there have been 21 general comments to date (2017).

In 2006, a General Comment on the Rights of Children with Disabilities was drafted and adopted:

- It specified in relation to Article 31 that children with disabilities have a right to access recreation activities appropriate to their age, and capability, including mental and psychological ability;

- That children with disabilities should be provided with equal opportunities, places, and time to play with each other (children with and without disabilities).

Strengthening the policy context: Play for Children with Disabilities - the UNCRPD, 2008

It is of note that every convention developed by the United Nations is intended to be used in conjunction with or complimentary to existing legislation and conventions. This is the case with Article 31 from the UNCRC, which needs also to be viewed in conjunction with the second significant convention: the Convention on the Rights of People with Disability (UNCRPD), which was developed by the United Nations and came into force in 2008. Although not aimed specifically at children, it contains articles that refer directly to children with disabilities, e.g.:

- Article 7 - States Parties shall take all necessary measures to ensure the full enjoyment by children with disabilities of all human rights and fundamental freedoms on an equal basis with other children;

- Article 26 - Support participation and inclusion in the community and all aspects of society, are voluntary, and are available to persons with disabilities as close as possible to their own communities, including in rural areas;

- Article 30 - To ensure that children with disabilities have equal access with other children to participation in play, recreation and leisure and sporting activities, including those activities in the school system.

Strengthening the policy context: Play for Children with Disabilities - General Comment No. 17, 2013

The most influential General Comment however for the rights of children to play, has been General Comment no 17 (GC17), which was adopted in 2013.

From the review process of the implementation of the UNCRC, the GC17 realised that states still had poor recognition of the right to play, resulting in poor investment, limited progress in legislation and policy, and 'invisibility of children in national and local-level planning'. They noted that when investment was made into play provision, it over-emphasised structured and organised activities rather than recognising the need to provide time and space for children. Specifically, the GC17 identified groups of children who were at risk of play deprivation more than others: these included children with disabilities. For children with disabilities the GC17 identified many barriers to play including: physical barriers - inaccessible playspaces and transport, policies that exclude participation on the grounds of safety, communication barriers, poor investment in technologies, and lack of involvement of children in designing for play.

With these concerns in mind, the CG17 went on to provide guidance on how to progress implementation of the UNCRC more effectively. Some key issues addressed include:

1. Creating a context for the realisation of Article 31 - including factors for an optimal environment;

2. Challenges to addressing the realisation of Article 31, including

- Lack of recognition of importance of play;
- Unsafe/hazardous environments;
- Resistance to children's use of public space;
- Balancing risk and safety;
- Lack of access to nature;
- Pressure for educational achievement;
- Overly structured schedules for children;
- Neglect of Article 31 in development programmes;
- Lack of investment in cultural and artistic opportunities;
- Growing role of electronic media;
- Commercialisation of play;

3. States parties obligations, covering aspects such as non-discrimination, and regulation, e.g.:

- 'public awareness of both the right to and the significance of play';
- 'establishment of safety and accessibility standards for all play and recreational facilities, toys and games equipment';
- 'all measures at local and national levels, and including planning, design, development, implementation and monitoring should be developed in collaboration with children themselves, as well as NGOs and community-based organisations';

- **Data collection and research:** 'States need to collect population-based data, disaggregated by age, sex, ethnicity and disability to gain an understanding of the extent and nature of children's engagement in play';

- **Universal Design:** 'investment in universal design is necessary with regard to play [...] consistent with obligations to promote inclusion and protect children with disabilities from discrimination';

- **Municipal planning:** local municipalities should assess provision of play and recreation facilities to guarantee equality of access by all groups of children and should include:

- **Availability of inclusive parks and playgrounds;**

  - Design of zones for free play;

  - Public safety measures to protect areas for play;

  - Access to green areas and nature for play;

  - Physical environments for play in schools designed for equal opportunity.

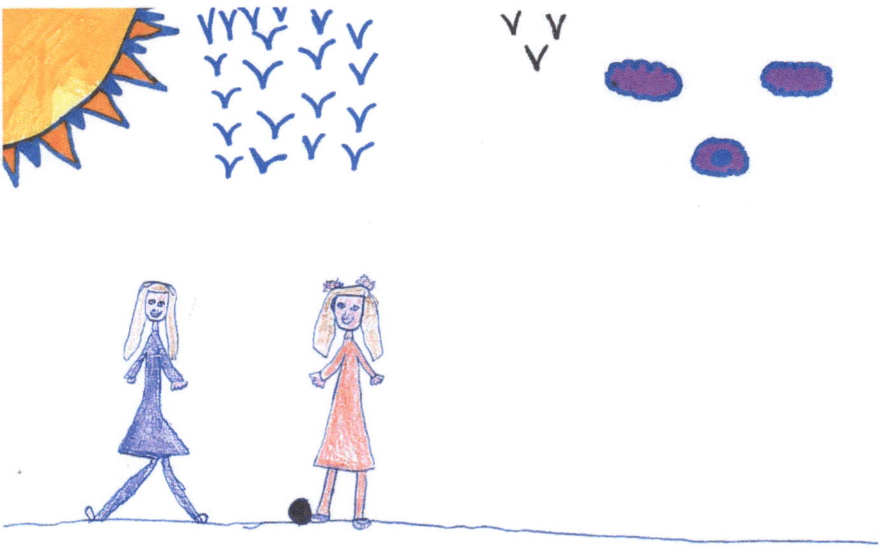

Rebecca, 8 years old, Italy

Case Study: The play sufficiency duty, Wales

Wales became the first country in the world to legislate for children's play by implementing a play sufficiency requirement that was informed by the UNCRC. The Children and Families (Wales) Measure 2010, Section 11 placed a statutory duty on every local authority to assess and secure sufficient play opportunities for children and young people in play areas. The play sufficiency duty came about as part of the Welsh Government's anti-poverty agenda, which recognises that children can have a poverty of experience, opportunity, and aspiration, and that this kind of poverty can affect children from all social, cultural, and economic backgrounds across Wales. Supporting improved access to play for children with disabilities was included in the second part of the play sufficiency duty. To support the introduction of this duty, the Welsh Government published Statutory Guidance and a Play Sufficiency Assessment Toolkit to support local authorities in fulfilling their duties.

Finally, more recently two key position statements have been published to further the play agenda for children with disabilities:

1. The International Play Association in 2015 published a Position Paper on the Play Rights of Disabled Children to further promote awareness and consciousness in the general public about the need to recognise this as a serious concern;

2. The LUDI COST Action produced its position statement in 2017.

Conclusion

Although play is a right enshrined in international conventions such as the United Nations Convention on the Rights of the Child and the United Nations Convention on the Rights of Persons with Disabilities, children with disabilities still face many barriers to play. These include the lack of political commitment to implementing the right to play, different values and attitudes in the socio-cultural environment, and inaccessible physical environment.

While it is a sad fact, it seems that as a society, we need to advocate for children's play: to give children permission to play, to promote play more in families of children with disabilities, to redress the imbalances identified in these policies. The emphasis on the future child (working always to develop skills that are perhaps delayed in development) needs to shift to include looking at the child in the here-and-now. Focus on current play needs will help future resilience and well-being. It is reassuring that from our review of policy, we have strong guidance on how to do this. Through work of networking organisations such as LUDI, the future for play for children with disabilities is very hopeful.

4

Are our children playing?

Daniela Bulgarelli and Francesca Caprino

How can we be sure that children are actually playing?

In Chapter 1, play has been defined, following Garvin, as 'a range of voluntary, intrinsically motivated activities normally associated with recreational pleasure and enjoyment'. Characteristics of play include intrinsic motivation, process oriented, enjoyment and pleasure, active engagement and internal control, and suspension of reality. Therefore, when assessing if a child is actually playing, one may ask several questions, addressing the different traits of play: are they having fun? Are they fully involved in the activity? Are they in charge of the activity? Can they choose what to do? Can they control their behaviours and the outcomes of their activities? Are they free to change and adapt their behaviours to meet their final ludic goals?

If you are used to play with children with disabilities and to observe them playing, you know that some of these questions are hard to answer. Yet, play assessment is crucial for several reasons: to help families supporting their children's right to play, to promote children's full inclusion in a wider range of play activities, to make informed decisions about educational and therapeutic programs aiming at developing and facilitating play. In line with the play definition above, this chapter addresses play assessment, and not 'play-based' assessment: in the first case, play is the focus; in the latter case, play is used as a means to evaluate other competences in children, as cognitive functioning, emotion regulation, social abilities, physical competences.

Play is a multidimensional construct and several aspects contribute to ludic activities. Thus, when adults wish to assess play, they need to identify which aspects to focus on and why, and then select the methodology of assessment.

Reasons to assess play, which aspect of play to assess and how to assess it

In the first place, the adult has to identify the aims to be achieved through play assessment. Possible goals include:

- To assess the child's strengths and weaknesses in play;

- To assess the child's needs in play: which activities can be proposed? In which moment of the day? In which context? Which features should have the playspaces? Which toys to choose? Which play partners?

- To assess the child's preferences in play: play materials and toys, games and play activities;

- To monitor the child's progress in play.

The second step consists in choosing which is the play dimension to focus on from:

- Types of play – the adult can assess the cognitive dimension of play (practice, symbolic, constructive and rule play) or the social dimension (solitary, parallel, associative and cooperative play);

- Play developmental stages – each type of play usually emerges in a specific period of life. Practice, solitary and parallel play are typical activities of the first year; symbolic, constructive, parallel and associative play emerge at about 18-24 months; children of about 3 years get involved in first forms of rule and co-operative play. As the children's competences grow, these types of play become more complex. They are also often mixed. For instance, 'hide and seek' shows features of practice, rule and cooperative play;

- Playfulness – this is the child's disposition to play. A playful child is internally motivated to play, is in control of the activities and its outcomes, is able to modulate the reality restrictions on the activity and is able to keep on going the interactions with the play partners. Therefore, playfulness partly depends on the child's characteristics, and partly depends on the environmental factors;

- Participation in play – full participation implies five aspects: a) the child attends and pays attention to play; b) he/she is involved in play; c) the child's preferences are addressed in the play activity; d) he/she is in the condition of exercising or improving his/her own competences in play; e) the play activity contributes to positively support or change self-confidence;

- Play contexts and environments – contextual factors refer to both space, objects, materials and to people's opinions, attitudes, knowledge, culture, etc. Different contexts (neighbourhood playgrounds, outdoor play areas, home, schoolyards, educational services, rehabilitative settings) involve different spaces, objects, materials, people, types of relationship, routines, habits that affect play in several ways.

Depending on the number and types of dimensions of play to evaluate, the assessment process will be more or less detailed.

The third step is deciding how to assess play. Different methodologies can be used:

- Interviews or questionnaires, addressed to the child or to other persons informed about his/her play activities, play preferences, etc.;

- Direct observation;

- Assessment tests. In this case, tests are usually designed to evaluate types of play or play stages.

Observation is considered the best method for assessing children's play as it provides a deeper understanding of children's behaviours in the context of everyday life and allows gathering direct information even with very young children or with children with communication impairments. Moreover, both professionals and non-professionals can assess play through observation. It is important to underline that more than one single methodology can be chosen to assess play. For example, the play observation could be preceded by a parent's interview.

Observing play

Observing should not be confused with casual looking. Observing means carefully watching with a critical and scientific attitude to acquire new knowledge. It is a data collection process in which the human observer is the tool to measure and collect the data.

It is worth noticing that observation always includes a subjective point of view on reality, because our interpretation of situations and behaviours is guided by our implicit theories. It is well known, for example, that Eskimos have about fifty words to describe the snow: their way to conceptualize snow is different from that of European people. Thus, an Eskimo and an Italian person watching the same snow will notice and describe different things. This process affects also people who watch children playing: they will focus on different aspects according to the idea of what a child is (a sort of little adult with inadequate abilities, a person who has to be taught, a competent person to listen to; etc.) and what play is (having fun, learning, travelling to an imaginary dimension, waste of time, occupation, childish activity, etc.) For this reason, before observing play, it is crucial to bring into awareness our implicit definition of play and its several aspects: this is necessary to be able to observe and describe more precisely what we are watching. Having more than one single observer can be another useful strategy to minimize the observer's bias.

For a successful data collection through observation, one should have present what to look at. Ad hoc checklists or available play assessment tools can support the observer. Depending on the observation methodology adopted (e.g. use of an observation tool), the observer can participate to the play activity (fully or partially) or have an onlooker role. The ideal contexts to observe play are the familiar ones, such as playgrounds, home or classrooms. In those places, children usually feel comfortable and safe, because they are surrounded by relatives and friends, everyday objects and familiar routines.

The presence of severe and/or multiple disabilities can make it harder to observe and evaluate play behaviours. Thus, it is worth noticing that the effective involvement in play can be expressed through non-verbal signals that offer multiple cues to understand children's internal states, even in those with multiple disabilities: facial expressions (smiling, eyes widening, eye flashing, eye gazing), vocalizations (laughing, giggling), body movements (jumping, doing vivacious hand gestures such as hands clapping or hands waving). Even in presence of severe physical impairments, it is possible to observe enjoyment and engagement in play. The authentic play experience is always associated with positive emotions such as joy, excitement, curiosity, interest, satisfaction, laughter. Moreover, every child shows some kind of play ability, even at basic levels. Children unable to engage in symbolic or make believe play, or who cannot use toys in a functional way (e.g. cannot throw a ball or pile bricks), may show very simple practice play abilities such as manipulating and exploring objects. Children may not display cooperative play behaviours but be able to play alone or just close to other children without interacting with them.

How to choose a tool to assess play

To support a systematic play assessment, it is possible to choose among a wide range of tools; some of them use direct sources of information (i.e., play observation), others use indirect sources, such as interviews and questionnaires, addressed to the children or to adults who are familiar to the child.

Using a tool to support play assessment through observation can be useful for several reasons:

- The authors of the tools have precisely described which aspect of play to assess;
- If the tool is validated, i.e. if it was verified that the tool does in fact measure what it is supposed to measure, one can rely on the outcome of the assessment;
- Results of assessments in different moments in time using the same tool are comparable to each other.

Tools can be standardized or not. In the context of assessment tools, standardisation refers to the following three concepts:

- Uniformity of the administration and scoring procedures – some tools require that all children are observed in similar conditions, using the same materials, proposing the same activities, etc. Additionally, the procedures to calculate the score are also precisely explained and should be precisely followed;

- Results are to be compared with a norm – a large number of children, divided into age groups (e.g. 5-year-olds, 6-year-olds, etc.) have been assessed using the tool and their scores were used to set the typical score of a child in a given age group. These typical scores and their standard deviations are called norms of the tool. The norms are reported in the manual or in the scientific paper describing the tool.

- Results are standardized – when using a tool to assess a competence, every child is attributed a raw score. The raw score is transformed into a standardised score to express how the child's score compares with the typical score of his/her age group. One way of computing standardized scores is using the formula

$$\text{Standardized score} = \frac{\text{raw score - average score of the age group}}{\text{standard deviations}}$$

In this case, a standardized score ranging from –1 to +1 means the child's performance is typical for his/her age; a standardized score lower than –2 means the child's performance is considerably lower than what is typical for his/her age; a standardized score higher than +2 means the child's performance is considerably higher than what is typical for his/her age. Another way of computing a standardized score is through

$$\text{Standardized score} = \frac{\text{raw score}}{\text{average score of the age group}} \times 100$$

Now, a standardized score ranging between 85 and 115 means typical performance for age; standardized scores lower than 75 mean considerable lower performance for age; and standardized scores higher than 130 mean consider able higher performance for age.

Standardized tools usually were validated and thus should be preferred over non-standardized tools.

Other factors that should be considered when choosing a tool to support play assessment through observation include:

- Which aspect of play is being assessed (play preferences, play activities, playfulness, environmental context, play opportunities, etc.);

- Who will be applying the tool – check if the tool is intended to be administered by clinicians or rehabilitation professionals (i.e., occupational therapists, speech and language therapists, psychologists, etc.), or by educators or non-professionals. Usually, this information is reported in the manual or in the scientific paper describing the tool, or it can be inferred by the professional context in which the tool has been developed;

- Tool's target group – check which is the group of people targeted by the tool (e.g. age range, country or culture of belonging, typically developing children and/or children with specific disabilities). Most of the formal assessment tools and methodologies are not specifically addressed to children with disabilities, although many of them have been tested on this target–group as well. Consequently, in some cases, the tool materials (e.g. the toys) or the testing procedures might be unsuitable for some children.

Once you have identified an assessment tool, it is possible that some adaptations of materials and/or procedures are necessary to be able to apply it to a particular group of children. Examples of adaptations include extending the time devoted to play, prompting the child, or providing physical support. Though these adaptations might be the only way of effectively applying the tool, keep in mind that they violate the standardization criteria and thus the tool's results should be used with caution.

In Chapter 11 you can find a list of available play assessment tools. Generally speaking, it is important to focus on several aspects of play: children's functioning, features of spaces and toys, characteristics of play partners, etc. The broader the view, the more informative and useful the assessment. Accordingly, it might be useful to use together two or more tools evaluating different aspects of play. For instance, the Test of Playfulness and the Test of Environmental Supportiveness were designed to be used together, the first to assess the child disposition to play and the second to assess the contextual features (e.g. spaces, materials, play partners, sensory environment) that enable or prevent play.

Assessing play: an ongoing process

Play is a dynamic activity and children's play change over time: for these reasons, play assessment is meant to be an ongoing process. It should point out the actual competences of the child, but also look at the potential of the child. This means that play assessment should address what children can do by themselves and what they can do with a certain degree of assistance provided by an adult or by a more expert peer. This is what the soviet psychologist Vygotsky called 'the zone of proximal development', the area of learning which occurs when some kind of help is offered to the child by a person with higher competences.

Given that play assessment is an ongoing process, it is worth noticing that it can be performed in a formal or informal way. Formal assessment refers to a specific and defined time dedicated to observe play, using the methodologies that have been already described. However, informal assessment of play, by observing frequently and regularly everyday episodes and events in a more flexible way, is also necessary and useful. For example, it allows tracking the child's advances in play, possibly due to educational or rehabilitative play interventions, and it can be a starting point to decide for a formal assessment or to decide which kind of formal assessment would be preferable.

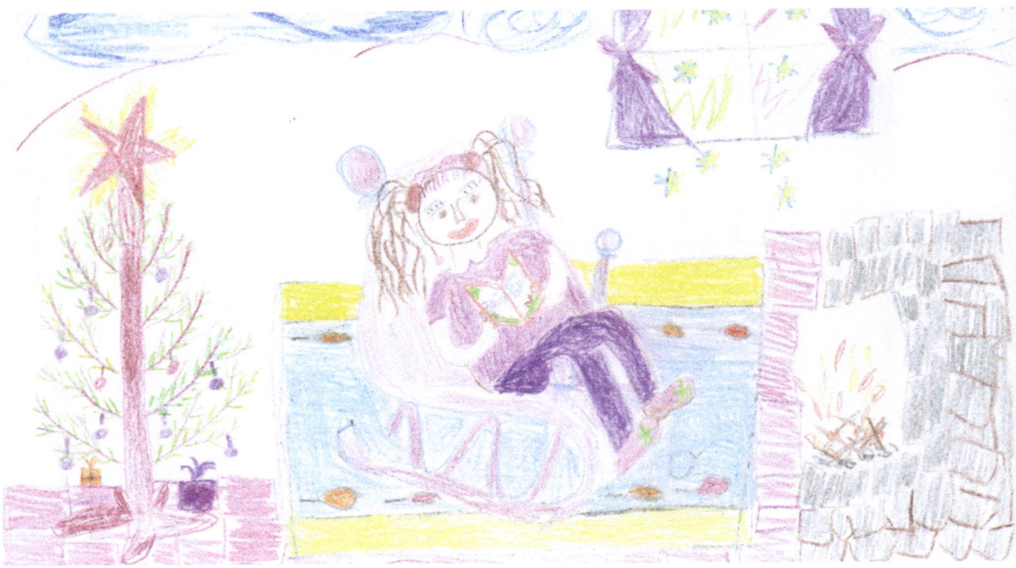

Elizabet, 6 years old, Bulgaria

Conclusion

The assessment of play is a powerful tool for the adults who want to facilitate play for the sake of play in children with disabilities: a deeper knowledge of the child's preferences, strengths and weaknesses is the basis of any intervention aimed at supporting play.

Play assessment is not meant to measure children's abilities; rather its goal is to collect the necessary information to better create the conditions such that children can play. Most importantly, play assessment is not a goal in itself, done to label a particular child in relation to some standard, it is a tool that should be used to help children being playful and widening their play opportunities.

5

How can I, as an adult, facilitate play?

Nicole Bianquin[1]

Adults have a crucial role in children's play

The literature highlights the fact that children learn to play: they usually learn by themselves with self-initiated play activities or imitating others in inclusive play situations, but sometimes they need adult's support.

Play for the sake of play can also be learnt.
An educator, a therapist or a parent can take part of the child's play to improve, increase, and develop it. The role of the adult should be limited to pursuing objectives inherent to the play itself, not turning play into a play-like activity for reaching external goals, other than recreational pleasure and enjoyment.

This awareness is not yet clearly shared. Often adults (parents or professionals) exert too much control over the child's play. Reasons for that include: a) over-protection; b) giving priority to interventions with educational or therapeutic purposes; c) discomfort or disapproval of the children's play; d) reduced expectations on independent activity of the child, motivated for example by a perceived low initiative and/or long child's reaction times; and e) underestimation of the value of play, considered as a waste of time and unproductive activity. Taking part of a child's play should be about playing with the child, fully aware of one's own adulthood

1 The author would like to thank Dr. Daniela Bulgarelli and Dr. Fabio Sacchio for their input on this text.

and educational competence, but maintaining and respecting the constraints and limitations of play itself and taking action to consolidate it, change it, and increase its complexity and flexibility as play, not as a means for learning or development.

When children with disabilities are involved, adult's intervention in play is even more important, as extensively shown by international research. Without adults' assistance, play often unfolds at lower levels for children with disabilities. However, with the careful and appropriate support from adults, play can move through naive play situations towards increasingly complex and challenging play situations. The adult's role in this process is of the utmost importance: parents, educators and therapists must learn how to teach children play. This involves a knowledge that is not innate nor embedded in the cultural repertoire. For example, adults must learn:

- How to teach children to use their body, with specific capabilities and limitations, in order to find pleasure and enjoyment in play;
- How to stimulate imagination, intellectual challenges, and relationships with others;
- How to set up the context to promote play (e.g. help the child to find a comfortable and functional play position, make the space welcoming and play appropriate, select the appropriate toys);
- How to apply specific play intervention techniques and methodologies; or
- How to use available advanced technology to facilitate and/or assess play.

The guiding principle is that any intervention to promote play must identify the child's characteristics and allow sufficient flexibility, unpredictability and safety for children to play. Adults' interventions should aim for creating an environment that supports children to choose freely what to do and how to do it. We hope that the present publication will guide an adult willing to acquire these competencies in his/her journey.

Becoming a builder of rights

All adults have responsibility for children's play, whether they are parents, educators, therapists, policy makers, or simply a fellow human being. Adults should be aware of the importance of play, play for the sake of play and not play with secondary goals, and promote and protect the conditions that support it. When interacting with children, adults should adopt a **playful framework**, both mentally and physically, provide dedicated time and space to play, and respect children's own play preferences, desires and needs. The adult in this context becomes a builder of rights. By granting the child the right to play, the main dimension of every child's life, he is recognising the right to childhood and the right to belong to a society that respects and welcomes the typical actions of children, and their contribution and approach to social life.

Becoming a promoter of inclusive play

Research studies show that children with disabilities have a desire to take part of the children's world. Playing with other children is the way to enter that world. The first challenge is to overcome social and attitudinal barriers. Adults need to understand the importance of play for every child and the benefits of an inclusive setting for all children. For example, a typically developing child, when used to model exemplary behaviours to his/her peers with disabilities, is likely to show increased self-esteem, confidence, autonomy and leadership skills. Adults should not overlook providing inclusive play opportunities to children with disabilities. These can happen indoor or outdoor, whenever more than one child meet together, for example in birthday parties, family reunions or an afternoon walk to the park. Inclusive play is instrumental to children with disabilities for making friends, experiencing childhood, and becoming a full member of the society. A child with enough inclusive play opportunities will learn how to manage conflicts and will be able to move between different social groups, expanding his/her capacity to communicate. Often adults are called to facilitate play, mediating interactions and constructing relationships between children, so they can learn to play together. They should however try to intervene as little as possible, allowing children to discover each other.

Becoming a scaffolder

When facilitating play, the adult's goal should be to guide and support children with disabilities in a path that leads them to acquire the skills and abilities necessary to become an expert in play for the sake of play, creating the environmental conditions that are most suitable for the functioning of that child, overcoming architectural, social and personal barriers. In this role, an adult is a **scaffolder**, a person who erects scaffolding. Scaffolding is placed around the outside of buildings under construction allowing builders to access the emerging structure as it rises from the ground. Once the building is able to support itself, the builder removes the scaffolding.

> The metaphor of **scaffolding** refers to the temporary support provided for learners to help them complete a task they would otherwise not be able to complete on their own. Effective scaffolding is tuned to the actual needs of learners, being constantly adjusted in response to their achievements, gradually fading away as they acquire the necessary skills.

Fundamental to the scaffolding methodology is the ability of identifying the child emotional and communication signals and appropriately respond to them, thus enabling a meaningful and effective interaction. The adult can assume three different main roles in facilitating and supporting play for children with disabilities: 1) Observer; 2) Activator; and 3) Partner. The adult will dynamically change his/her role and change the interaction with the child accordingly.

Adult as Observer

The first role of an adult when facilitating play is that of an Observer. The goal is to identify the child play skills and what he/she would like to do. It is essential to gather information about the child himself (e.g. desires, needs, degree of autonomy, attention, concentration) and about the child's play (e.g. play preferences, degree of playfulness, recurring or missing play typologies) in order to be able to build play situations that are appropriate for the particular child. In this process, the adult must be aware that his observations are always influenced by the models of play and of education that are present in his memory. It is therefore important to internalize the concept of play: 'a range of voluntary, intrinsically motivated activities normally associated with recreational pleasure and enjoyment'.

Although parents have an in-depth knowledge of their children, they should not neglect the need of purposely observing their children in order to understand how they play, with what, with whom, and also with what and with whom they would like to play. Professionals as well should take the time necessary to observe and get to know the child. Numerous tools are available today to support play observations, assessing for example the play autonomy, the levels of playfulness, or the play typologies (see Chapter 4 for more details).

Adult as Activator

The adult in the role of Activator should identify the best promising conditions from which play can spring, exist and evolve. A so-called **playful framework** should be created. Taking into consideration the child characteristics and having in mind that play is the foundation of childhood, the activator dedicates space and time for the child to experience play for the sake of play. Playful and inclusive play situations need to be designed and suitable toys need to be chosen. The activator role involves several tasks, including:

- Organising or selecting play environments;
- Making time for play in the child and adult daily routines;
- Choosing and making available to the child appropriate toys;
- Planning and suggesting play activities that interest, intrigue and motivate the child;
- Fostering inclusion, e.g. creating play situations that naturally result in physical contact between children with and without disabilities.

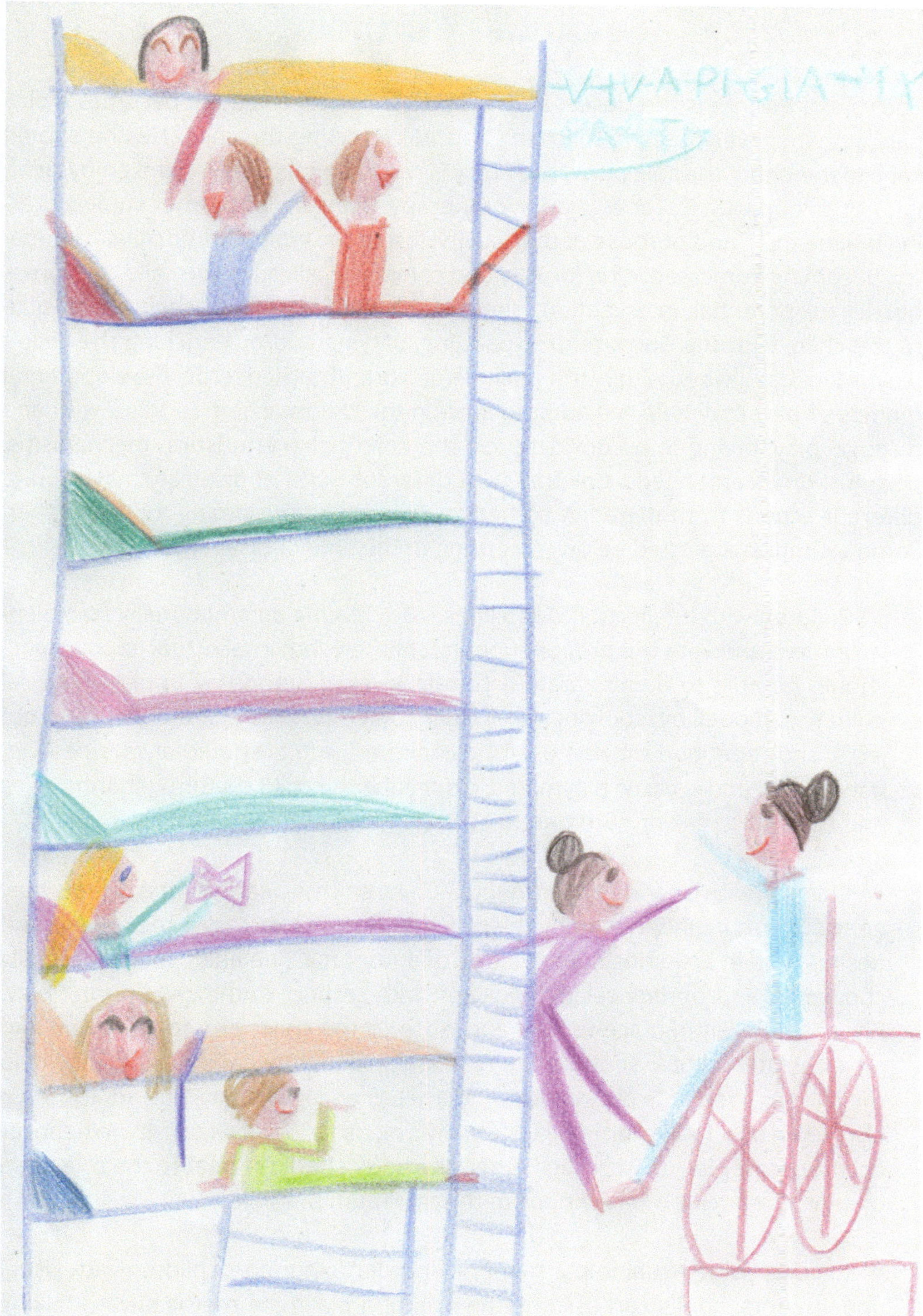

Arianna, 7 years old, Italy

Adult as Partner

The role of Partner is the closest to that of a scaffolder. The adult becomes a play partner, whenever possible following and not directing the child. He/she should keep in mind that the sole purpose of play is recreational pleasure and enjoyment; it is not an opportunity for education or therapy. Being a play partner implies sharing the meaning and purpose of the activity, losing the typical adult/child asymmetry, becoming immersed in reciprocity and complicity, allowing the child to express his/her full potential. Interventions should be limited to suggest changes, feasible to the child, with the purpose of expanding, varying and/or enriching the child's play interests, always within the play framework. Knowledge on developmental models of play may help the adult to sustain the child's action, to 'work with and through play' taking into consideration the child's characteristics, mechanisms, rhythms, times and needs. Children with different types of disability may require different actions from the adult so he/she succeeds in becoming a play partner. Some examples are listed below, according to the type of disability:

- Children with Intellectual Disabilities – By creating an emotionally stable environment and with the proper support, children with intellectual impairments should be able to demonstrate a certain level of autonomy in play. Physical guidance; modelling, showing concretely how to do things and how to use objects; and repetition may be useful techniques. Adults should always be kind, patient and enthusiastic playmates, respecting the child rhythms, sharing roles and rules, and making sure that the child is having fun.

- Children with Hearing Impairments – Children with hearing impairments may need support in understanding the play situation, in expressing their needs and desires, and in acquiring some degree of autonomy. The adult should carefully choose an appropriate relative position with respect to the child during play. For example, sitting face-to-face and close to the child, promoting visual and physical interactions, showing the toys and inviting the child to play, may help the child to overcome the barriers and actively engage in play. The adult should also serve as a facilitator of inclusion, inviting other children to play. Whenever children start playing with each other, the adult should retreat to the role of an observer, reducing interventions to the minimum possible.

- Children with Visual Impairments – In order to support children with visual impairments, adults can assume the role of a playmate that is always talking about what is happening, thus providing the necessary feedback on the play situation to the child. For example, in case of constructive play, frequent feedback on how construction is going can help the child to mentally represent the object being built and plan the necessary actions to finalize the project. When other children are involved, adults may mediate the relationships between the child with visual impairments and other children, thus ensuring that all children actively take part of play.

• Children with Communication Disorders – The essential task of adults, when playing with children with communication disorders, is to support and enrich children's language, enabling them to express their feelings, ideas, needs and requests. Enough time should be given for the child to convey his/her message, without constantly trying to guess what the child has to say. In addition, adults have a central role in promoting and facilitating inclusive play. They should help the child with communication disorders to understand the play situation and the playmates' proposals, but also help the other children in learning how to communicate with the child with communication disorders. The ultimate goal is to develop in all playmates the necessary communication skills such that play can happen without adult intervention.

• Children with Severe Physical Impairments – The adult playmate of a child with severe physical impairments should be very patient, allowing the necessary time for the child to complete an action by him/herself, resisting to the urge of substituting the child. The adult should provide opportunities for the child to play autonomously, regardless of his/her impairment, for example making use of adapted toys. In inclusive play situations, the adult should also pay attention to the other children, helping them in finding appropriate ways of interacting with the child with physical impairments, and promoting play activities in which all can take an active role.

• Children with Autism Spectrum Disorders – When playing with a child with Autism Spectrum Disorders, the adult needs to gain the trust of the child and design a play framework in which the child feels comfortable and safe. Adults should then gradually introduce novelties into the play situation. For example, one can take a story that is already familiar to the child and invite the child to play a role in it, then introducing some new elements. In the case of constructive play, the adult may model how to go on with the construction, preventing the child from always focusing on the same sequence. Special attention should be given to avoid or reduce frustrations, clearly explaining the play situations and providing support when needed. Additionally, adults should ensure that the sensorial characteristics of the play situation (lights, colours, sounds, objects, smells) are appropriate for the child.

- Children with Multiple Disabilities – Although sometimes extremely challenging, play is as fundamental for children with multiple disabilities as for any other child. Physical contact and continuous verbalization should be used to patiently explain, give meaning, encourage, and congratulate the child. Especially with these children, adults should build on their interests and preferences, proposing play activities that are of their interest and that they are able to perform, and then slowly increase the challenge to the child. Often play with these children involves repeated patterns of movement or sound (practice play) and only with the proper support from an adult it can evolve in variety and complexity.

Conclusion

Adults have a crucial role in children with disabilities' play. By clearly understanding the importance of play for the sake of play for all children, adults can become guardians of the children's right to play, ensuring them enough opportunities for playing by themselves and with others. In play situations, adults are called to support children. They should observe to understand the child play skills, preferences and needs; then they should activate play by creating a motivating play framework; finally, they should become play partners, always respecting the child's play preferences, providing only the needed support, and making sure that the play always contains the right amount of challenge to keep the child engaged. The metaphor of scaffolding is particularly enlightening: the adult should support the child while he/she is acquiring play skills in the same way scaffolding supports the construction of a new building. Once the child has acquired the necessary skills to play on his/her own, scaffolding should be removed.

6

What assistive technologies exist to enable participation in play?

Pedro Encarnação and Rianne Jansens

Participation in play often requires staying in a comfortable and functional position, moving around, manipulating objects, communicating, or using a computer or tablet. This chapter briefly refers to technologies that may reduce the gap between the requirements of the play and the children's abilities by providing support in the above general-purpose functional areas or by adapting the activity. Adapted toys and games are discussed in Chapter 7 and accessible digital games in Chapter 8.

What is Assistive Technology?

Following the World Health Organization definition, Assistive Technology 'is the application of organized knowledge and skills related to assistive products, including systems and services'. An Assistive Product is 'any external product (including devices, equipment, instruments or software), especially produced or generally available, the primary purpose of which is to maintain or improve an individual's functioning and independence, and thereby promote their well-being'.

The International Organization for Standardization (ISO) issued a classification of assistive products in its ISO 9999 international standard. This classification is widely used around the globe, especially for prescription of assistive products purposes. An overview of the different ISO 9999 classes can be obtained at the web page http://www.eastin.eu/en/searches/products/iso maintained by EASTIN. EASTIN is the European Assistive Technology Information Network offering information on assistive technology to all citizens. The network features the website http://www.eastin.eu where one can find, in all official languages of the European Union, and in a user-friendly and accessible manner, information and guidance tools on assistive technology. Over 70.000 assistive products (APs) are covered including practical information on assistive solutions for daily living problems.

Assistive products may be custom-made, satisfying the particular needs of a particular user (e.g. a custom contoured cushion); may be commercially available, having been developed for a generic user with a given condition (e.g. a wheelchair); or can be a mainstream technology developed for all (e.g. a computer or even Velcro® when used to help object manipulation). In reality, assistive products may lie in a continuum from custom-made to mainstream technology. For example, one can adapt a commercially available AP so it fits the particular needs of a user, thus lying between a commercially available and a custom-made assistive product. Mainstream assistive products are typically easier to obtain and less expensive than devices that are produced specifically for individuals with disabilities. However, it can be harder to obtain funding for mainstream products since funding programs often exclude those products to prevent abuse.

APs for seating and positioning

If not in a comfortable position that promotes function, a child is not able to play or interact. APs for seating and positioning serve three goals: postural control (ISO Code 09.07), tissue integrity (ISO Code 04.33), and comfort. Postural control is needed when children have impaired motor control such as abnormal muscle tone, muscle weakness, primitive reflexes or uncoordinated movements. Children that use a wheelchair and have limited ability to reposition themselves and/or do not sense pain or discomfort are at a risk of developing pressure ulcers, thus may need some assistance for keeping tissue integrity. For some children with mobility impairments, sitting for a long time causes discomfort from which they are unable to obtain relief. This discomfort may decrease their ability to participate in play. Technologies used to address the three goals above include seating systems like cushions, available in different materials with different properties, posture supports, belts, harnesses or straps to restrain uncontrolled movements or support the trunk and limbs for enabling fine motor movements. Postural control may also be facilitated with specific purpose benches or chairs, with non-standard dimensions and/or support components (e.g. head, arm, hip, or leg rests).

Children play in all kind of positions: standing, seated on the floor or on a chair, lying on their bellies or on their backs, knelt or crouched down, hanging from a sofa or bed, etc. They often change position while playing depending on the experienced comfort and in response to the demands of the task in relation to their abilities. This constitutes a challenge when considering seating and positioning APs to enable participation in play and frequently non-traditional solutions need to be adopted, along with adaptations to the playspace, in order not to spoil the play experience.

APs for mobility

Many times playing requires functional mobility, or participation is enhanced by being able to move independently. Children with mobility impairments may need only a cane, walker or crutch to support mobility (ISO Codes 12.03 and 12.06), but for more severe impairments, a wheelchair, manual (ISO Code 12.22) or powered (ISO Code 12.23), may be necessary. For outdoor play, pedal-propelled vehicles for two or more persons (ISO Code 12.18.15) can create play opportunities (e.g. enabling participation in a hide and seek game).

In the past, several concerns advised against the use of powered mobility by young children, including safety issues, acquisition and replacement costs, and possible detrimental effects on the development of self-locomotion. However, research in the last years supports the provision of powered mobility to children at an appropriate developmental time (the closest to when typically developing children start to walk as possible). Research also shows that training children on the use of a wheelchair should not be focused on learning how to control the wheelchair but rather on achieving functional goals (e.g. participating in a play-like activity) using the wheelchair.

APs for manipulation

Often play involves the manipulation of objects (e.g. toys), which may be challenging for children with physical impairments. APs for manipulation range from low-tech devices that facilitate grasping (ISO Code 24.18.03), reaching (ISO Code 24.21.03), or holding (ISO Code 24.18.09), to high-tech devices such as robotic manipulators (ISO Code 24.18.30) or prosthesis (ISO Code 06.18.24). Today, with 3D printing, it is possible to obtain an inexpensive functional prosthesis. Examples can be found in the platform Patient Innovation (https://patient-innovation.com/), a platform that shares solutions created by patients (or their carers) to help them coping with their day-to-day challenges. Lego® Mindstorms® robots (https://www.lego.com/en-us/mindstorms/) have also been used as manipulation tools enabling children to participate in play activities. Manipulation also includes operating and controlling devices. Push buttons (ISO Code 24.09.03) or switches (ISO Code 24.09.18) are examples of APs that may enable a child to control an electronic toy.

APs for communication

Communication is the very essence of being human and to be able to communicate with others is required for full participation in play, either to interact with playmates or with a play facilitator. Children with complex communication needs may use speech-generating devices (ISO Code 22.21.09) to produce voice output from a written text or by selecting an appropriate option in an augmentative and alternative communication (AAC) software.

Nowadays AAC software is available for mainstream technology such as iPads or smart phones. These might be preferable for children, provided that the child has the necessary fine motor and cognitive skills to use them, since the stigma associated to these devices is smaller. Communication via an AAC software is often slow, requiring the user to write the text to be spoken or to go through a set of selections. In play situations, this delay can hamper participation. Simple devices as switches that produce digitally recorded speech output upon a switch press may be a good alternative for some play scenarios (e.g. telling a story together where each child is responsible for the voice of a character; the character lines may be pre-recorded and the child only has to hit the switch when it is his/her turn). Other concerns when using AAC devices in play include making sure that appropriate vocabulary is available for the child and that the AAC system is mounted such that it does not get in the way of play.

Another way of addressing communication issues in play is to incorporate different forms of communication within the play objects. For example, parts of a toy/game can have different textures or contain braille text; tactile feedback may be provided in addition to auditory and/or visual feedback; visual information can include pictures, pictorial communication symbols, or sign language.

APs for accessing the computer or tablet

When using a computer, one has to provide inputs using the keyboard, a mouse, a touch screen, or another input system. That can be done by using a method to select directly the desired option among all the possible options. For example, one can directly select one letter in a computer keyboard, or use a mouse or a finger to directly select an option on a screen, or use the voice to indicate the choice. Direct selection is the fastest and easier selection method but requires refined and controlled movements. Input devices for direct selection (ISO Code 22.36) include keyboards (standard or modified), mice (standard or modified), eye tracking systems, or head pointers. When direct selection is impossible, the different options can be presented one at a time to the user that can select the desired with a single movement (e.g. pressing a switch). This is called indirect selection through scanning. It requires very little motor control but good visual tracking skills, a high degree of attention, and the ability to sequence. There is a great variety of switches (ISO Code 24.09.18) to support indirect selection (e.g. mechanical, electromagnetic, electrical control, proximity, pneumatic, or phonation switches). Special care should be given to the positioning of the input devices and routing of the cables, maximizing function and not interfering with the activity.

APs for seeing and hearing

Visual and auditory impairments may constitute a barrier to play. Anyone watching children playing will observe that visual information and sounds are an important part of any activity. Children with low vision can benefit from APs that augment their visual abilities such as lenses (ISO Code 22.03.09) or devices for displaying an enlarged image of the subject that has been captured by a video camera (ISO code 22.03.18). For blind persons, APs can provide alternative ways to convey visual information, translating visual inputs to tactile or auditory inputs. Examples are tactile computer displays (ISO Code 22.39.05) or screen readers (22.39.12).

Devices for concentrating, amplifying and modulating sound (ISO Code 22.06) may augment the hearing abilities of children with hearing loss. Voice to text software

(ISO Code 22.36.18) or sound indicators (ISO Code 22.27.18) provide alternative sensory pathways for deaf children that can be used in play situations.

APs for understanding the play situation

Sometimes play involves following rules, often set on the fly by playmates. When children play with toys, usually they attribute them different meanings and functions, varying over time. This can be challenging for a child with cognitive impairments. APs can help to keep track of instructions or time (ISO Codes 22.27.12, 22.27.15, 22.27.16 and 22.27.33). APs for marking and identifying materials (ISO Code 22.27.27) can be used to make clear different meanings of an object.

AAC products for face-to-face communication (ISO Code 22.21) and AAC techniques may be helpful to provide instructions about the play in an easy to understand way or to provide an overview of the activity that the child can refer back to when needed.

Play can involve many partners, be very dynamic and noisy, overwhelming children with different stimuli. A headphone (ISO Code 22.06.06) can help a child to focus and reduce stimuli.

Design for All

According to the Design for All Foundation (http://designforall.org/), 'Design for All [Universal Design] is the intervention into environments, products and services which aims to ensure that anyone, including future generations, regardless of age, gender, capacities or cultural background, can participate in social, economic, cultural and leisure activities with equal opportunities'. Design for All fosters user-centred design where the diverse needs of all are taken into account. A day-to-day example is elevator button panels with braille labels. The major computer, tablets and mobile phones operating systems have already built in accessibility functions. They include high contrast themes, a narrator that reads aloud any text on screen, a magnifier that zooms the area of the screen where the mouse is, changing the mouse cursor size and speed, on-screen keyboards, and voice-control. These are available through 'Ease of Access Centre' in Windows, 'Accessibility' options in iOS and Android. In some cases, they may be enough to make the device accessible for a particular child, thus avoiding the need of additional assistive technology.

The process of choosing an AP

Choosing an Assistive Product should be a user-centred process. It is the user, with his/her physical, cognitive and emotional characteristics, that wants to perform an activity, within a given physical, social, cultural and institutional context, that should have the final word in the choice of an AP to support him/her. This is also true for children, especially because their viewpoints on activities and assistive technology are often different from those of adults. For example, an AP might be fun and interesting to a child, but the stigma of its use may make it difficult for a parent to accept it for the child. Assessment for assistive technology should be made by a multidisciplinary team and be as comprehensive as possible, evaluating not only the needs of the particular client but also the context in which the AP will be used. Family members and significant others should be involved in the process since many times they will be co-users of the AP.

APs funding

In Europe, each country's social insurance or tax system finance assistive technology. Often public funding of assistive technology is described in relevant social legislation. For example, in some countries, lists of assistive products that are financed by public funds are published. It is worth mentioning that all European countries have signed the United Nations Convention on the Right of Persons with Disabilities and, with the exception of Ireland and Belarus, the Convention was already ratified by the national parliaments. Article 4 of this Convention forces the signatories to perform and promote research and development in assistive technology and design for all, and to make available accessible information on assistive technology. The great majority of the European countries also ratified the Optional Protocol to the Convention, enabling citizens to appeal to the Committee on the Rights of Persons with Disabilities when they believe they are victims of a violation by that country of the provisions of the Convention. Private insurances may also cover assistive technology expenses. Clinicians are aware of the requirements and of the process to apply for public and private funding and thus can assist the client in obtaining funding for assistive technology.

Conclusion

Play is a very diverse activity. Children play on their own or with others, with or without objects. Their play may be boisterous or quiet, light-hearted or very serious. By definition, play is an activity for enjoyment and recreation, without a practical purpose, which can make it hard to understand for those not participating in it. Therefore, requirements of play can also be very diverse. They may require a child to stand still quiet or to move around; to communicate with others or to understand and follow instructions; to manipulate objects or access a computer.

There are many Assistive Products than can enable participation of a child with disabilities in play, either by supporting children in some functional task, or by adapting the task such that it becomes accessible to a particular child. When selecting an AP to support play, the characteristics of the play need to be taken into consideration such that the AP does not come in the way of fun and enjoyment. Take your time exploring the EASTIN database for choosing an AP. The ISO Codes provided in this chapter may guide your search. Many times one needs to think out of the box, adapting APs that were mainly developed for other purposes. Be creative!

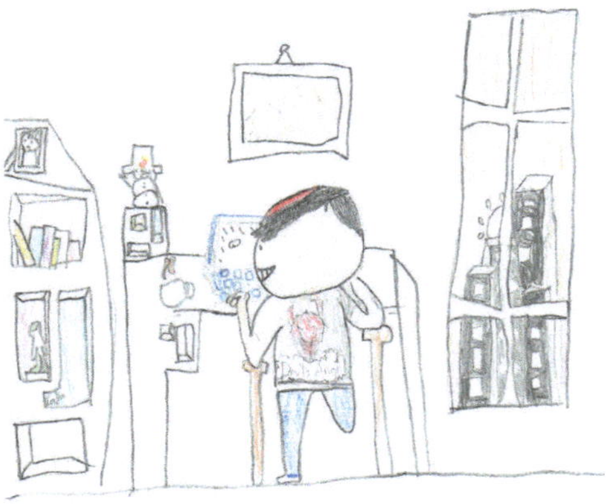

Daniel, 10 years old, Malta

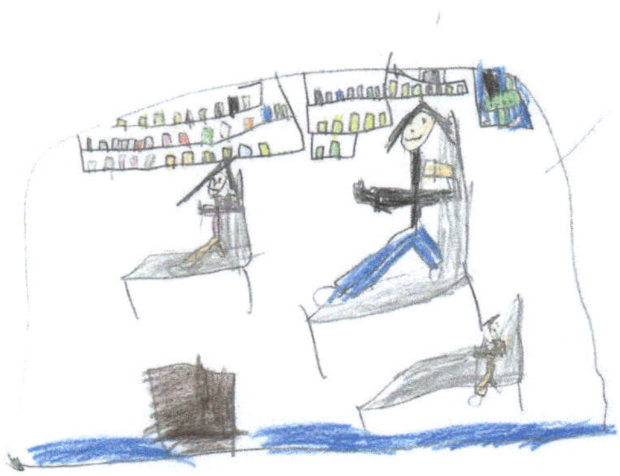

Aiden, 6 years old, Malta

7

Which toys and games are appropriate for our children?

Sylvie Ray-Kaeser, Odile Perino, Maria Costa, Eleanor Schneider, Vardit Kindler and Andrea Bonarini

Toys and games

Mainstream toys are 3-Dimensional and sensorial objects that adults give children to support their play activities and which are designed with this intention.

Although toys are the tools of play, play is not an attribute of toys. The play belongs to the player, to the child who wants and needs to play as long as the toy is compatible with his/her functioning and interests.

However, any object can become a toy if the child chooses to play with it and if the safety conditions are guaranteed. For example, a toy can be an object from nature (e.g. pebbles, leaves) or an object from the house (e.g. pan, adult shoe, empty box, paper).

Toys belong to the concrete reality where a child lives. They are essential mediators between a child and his/her environment. They are means for social exchange between children and enable them to play together. Being a mediator between the physical reality and its symbolic representation, toys also empower a child to express his/her feelings, worries or concerns.

In recent years, and thanks to electronics, a more subtle mechanism of interaction has been introduced in some toys. It is possible to add sensors that can perceive actions, so that the toy can autonomously react with varying degrees of complexity while maintaining its characteristics. The resulting interaction may enable a different relationship with the toy, not only as an object that can be used at the player's will, or can do exactly what the player wants, but also as an agent that can decide to do what it 'wants'. These toys may provide other play challenges, where the player has to understand how the toy is behaving and adapt his/her activity to that of the toy.

Games are a structured and competitive form of play. Key components of games are rules, which should be understood, freely accepted and followed by the players. Most games involve more than one player, thereby encouraging development of social relationships. Games generally involve mental or physical stimulation, and often both.

In many situations, a game is supported by objects, instrumental to the game, such as cards, a rope, a ball or a computer. The gaming situation can also be abstract as in word games.

Toys and games should be chosen according to the capacities and interests of the play participants in order to enable them to experience playfulness.

There are toys or games for the different types of play:

- Toys for practice play – sensorial toys or toys to manipulate and experiment with the body and encourage experiencing 'cause and effect' (e.g. rattles, toys to squeeze, empty and fill, push toys).

- Toys for symbolic play – toys used to imitate or simulate a situation and play scenario (e.g. a sword, a doll, a kitchen-set).

- Toys for constructive play – toys to assemble, combine and arrange, create (e.g. blocks).

- Games with rules – games to achieve intended objectives by following the rules of the play (e.g. board games, strategy games, video games).

Ideas of recommended toys by play types

Toys for practice play e.g. 'Pull along Gussy' from Andreu Toys

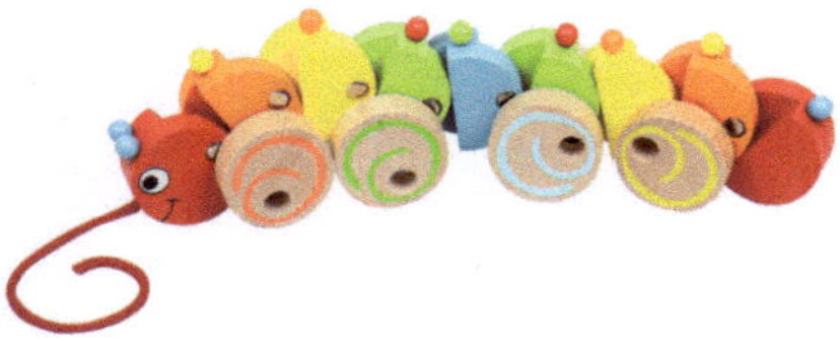

Photo used with permission.

Toys for symbolic play e.g. anatomically correct doll from Miniland; Parking Garage from PlanToys®

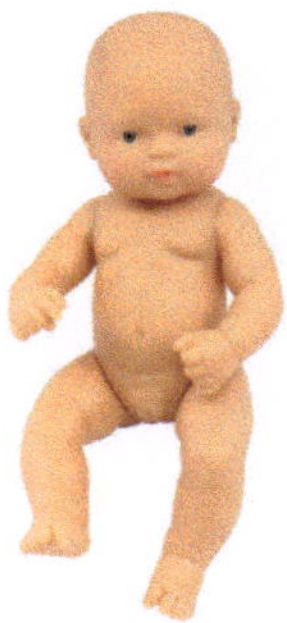

Photo used with permission.

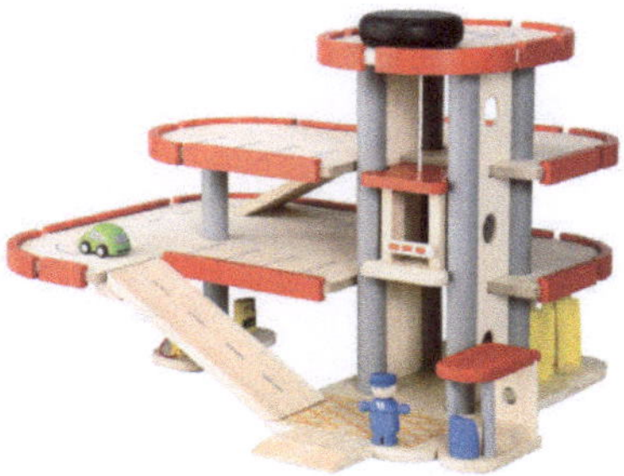

Photo used with permission.

Toys for constructive play e.g. building bricks from Lego®

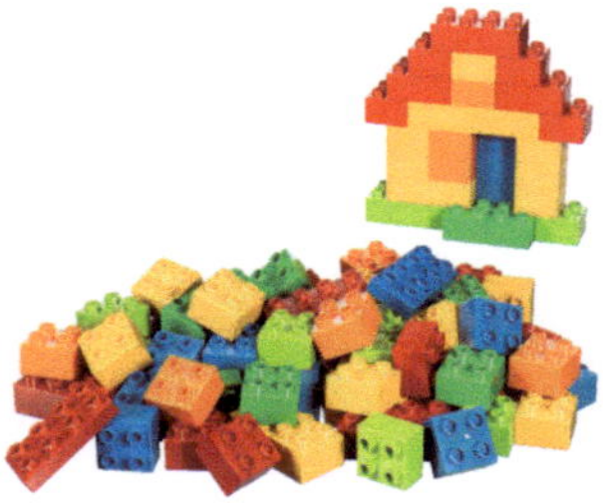

Photo used with permission. ©2018 The LEGO Group.[2]

Games with rules e.g. family cooperative game from Haba®

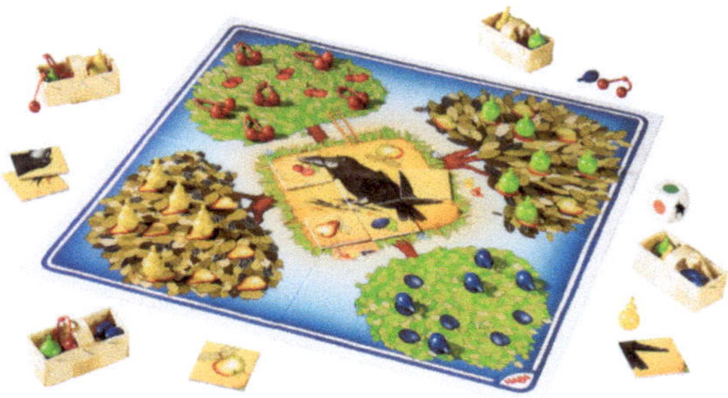

Photo used with permission. ©Habermaass GmbH

[2] All information is collected and interpreted by its authors and does not represent the opinion of the LEGO Group.

Accessible toys and games for all

All children differ in their functioning and preferences. Toys and games are **accessible** when they can be used by all children and when their different components are suitable for all abilities. **Inclusive toys and games** promote play exchanges between children with different skills and offer the possibility for them to feel a sense of belonging to the community of children players.

Certain elements embedded into the design of toys and games will allow more children to successfully interact and play with them. In order to design a flexible, adjustable, usable toy, multiple options must be present.

Universal Design is a philosophy for designing products that are usable by people with the widest possible range of functional capacities. The more Universal Design features a toy or game has, the more likely it is that it can be used successfully by a broad range of children, including those with disabilities. The general principles of Universal Design can be broadly defined as multiple means of representation, multiple means of use and multiple means of play. Below is a selection of the main principles:

- Toys and games should be accessible, flexible and adjustable.

- Toys and games should offer multiple means of play to be an open source of experiences.

- Toys and games should appeal to children with different abilities, encouraging exploration and discovery.

- Toys and games should offer easy ways to use them successfully.

- The overall structure and pieces of the toy/game should feature usable shapes, dimensions and weights: stable, big, light, allowing it to be grasped in different ways, etc.

- Toys and games should be able to be used in different positions, or be disassembled in modules in order to adjust them to the child.

- Toys and games should promote interactive actions and stimulate multisensory and multimodal experiences.

- Toys and games should have multiple sensory effects: sounds, lights, pictures, movements, vibrations, scents, textures, colours.

- Toys and games should include adjustable features for sound, height and level of difficulty to adapt to individual users.

- Toys and games should offer written and/or audible messages to adapt to individual user capabilities.

- Toys and games should have a quick and simple means of activation: one that does not require many steps in order to begin play.

- The toy and game components as well as buttons, switches, etc., should be easy to connect, to press, to turn on, fit in, grasp, etc.

- The activation buttons, knobs, connectors, etc., of the toy/game should be highlighted and differentiated from the background.

- The toy and game material should be washable.

In addition to these principles, each toy or game must meet safety standards as well as specific regional legal regulations. Finally, the toys/games should include other specific quality requirements, such as durability, comprehensibility, proper functioning as well as the potential for interaction and popularity, which are all aspects that children value.

Applying Universal Design concepts in the design process guarantees better use of the toy for most children and minimises the need for adaptations. For example, a ball with contrasting colours that vibrates and makes noises when rolled may be appropriate for children with a variety of disabilities including hearing or visual impairments and intellectual disabilities.

When designing a toy with sound signals, one must be sure that there is a volume control or other effects to enable a child with hearing impairments perceive the signals (lights, vibrations, written messages...).

When designing a toy with accessories or with many pieces, the latter should be sufficiently large, easy to assemble and multi-textured so that a child with visual or motor impairments can play with it.

Reviewing the physical characteristics of a toy can help families and caregivers make a decision about its accessibility for a specific group of children.

- Families can have more success in selecting toys for their children by identifying toys that have been designed with Universal Design concepts in mind. These designs not only address individual barriers, but also offer a combination of features to provide the greatest access to children of all abilities.

For ideas of toys accessible for any child:

AblePlay™ toy guide http://www.lekotek.org/images/stories/files/pdf/ableplay_toyguide_FINAL_web.pdf

AIJU toy guide http://www.guiaaiju.com/

EASTIN database on assistive technology http://www.eastin.eu/en/searches/freetext/summary?freetext=toys

For the assessment of the usability of toys and games by children with hearing, visual or motor impairments:

The 'TUET - Toys and games Usability Evaluation Tool' developed within the LUDI COST Action. http://www.tuet.eu

Selecting toys and games

Well-chosen toys and games, when used in a suitable environment, in a playful context, with play partners, children or adults, have the best chance to allow all children to play for the sake of play.

When selecting a toy or a game for a child, it is important to consider the features of the toy or game, the child's abilities, needs and preferences, the activity promoted by the toy or game and the expected play context. Indeed, even with the best-designed toy or game, it is not guaranteed that a child can and will play. Although toys and games are designed to perform a specific activity, in principle they can be used for play in a variety of ways. When selecting a toy or a game, there is freedom to explore possible alternative ways to use it and reshape the corresponding activity or adapt the toy or game to match the abilities and preferences of the player.

- It is important to remember that the best toy is the one that matches the child's characteristics (skills and abilities, personal preferences) and the play characteristics (level of challenge, demands and requirements of the activity).

Selecting the optimal toy or game requires an analysis of both the child's abilities and preferences as well as an analysis of the toy or game and play itself.

Information can be obtained in two main ways:

a. By asking the child/caregivers questions in order to define a child's needs and preferences in relation to toys/games and level of ability/skill. It is also important to consider the caregivers' preferences and abilities in playing with the child.

b. By observing the child in different play situations looking at a variety of behaviours, using an informal or formal play evaluation when appropriate.

With regard to elements related to the child

- What toys does the child prefer and succeed at playing with, and consider fun and enjoyable?

- With whom does the child like to play – alone, with peers, siblings, parents, caregivers?

- What is the preferable play context for the child – indoors or outdoors, the positions for play - moving, sitting or lying?

- Does the child have time for play? Is there a preferred or optimal time during the daily routine? Does the child have time to enjoy and control the play with the toy?

- What toys/materials are available for the child to play with?

- Are there differences in the child's level of performance – persistence, attention, coordination, mobility, communication, wellbeing, enjoyment with different kinds of toys, play partners, play context?

With regard to elements related to the toy/activity

a. General aspects related to the toy/activity

- For what age group/developmental level is the toy/activity appropriate?

  ☞ There is an advantage in buying toys that can be used with children of different ages in different ways, for example: balls, building blocks, drawing materials.

- Is the toy typically associated with gender, culture (e.g. dolls, trucks, toys for cooking)?

  ☞ Lack of gender dependency is preferable to enable more varied use.

- What is the cost of the toy?

  ☞ If the toy can be used in a variety of ways and is multipurpose, it is likely to be more cost effective.

- Physical requirements: are any additional materials needed?

- What are the space requirements, large vs small space, level of noise, lighting? Is there room for adjustment?

- How much time is needed for playing with the toy? Can the play activity be broken up into smaller parts and completed over a reasonable period of time?

    ☞ This is a positive aspect.

- How many steps are required to play with the toy?

    ☞ There is an advantage in toys where there is the potential to modify or grade the steps, varying the level of required mediation in playing.

- Safety precautions: is there potential for physical harm, allergic reaction, or psychological distress?

- What skills are required and what can be facilitated?

- Is there potential for adaptation or modification of the toy to match the child's needs?

b. Specific aspects related to the toy/activity

Motor requirements

- What is the required position/posture? Can it be changed/modified?

- What mobility, range of movements, dexterity, bilateral hand use and coordination are required? What motor planning is required?

- What strength and endurance are required?

Sensory requirements

- What sensory input/feedback are required and provided – visual, auditory, touch/pain/temperature, vestibular, proprioceptive, olfactory, taste?

- What sensory discrimination is required?

Cognitive requirements

- How much attention span and concentration are needed? Memory? Planning? Problem solving? Level of arousal? Judgment? Understanding? Learning?

Perceptual requirements

- Does the toy demand identification or matching by size, colour, shape, quantity? Should the player be able to distinguish left from right? Are figure-ground perception, depth perception required?

- How much visual-perceptual-motor integration is required?

Social-emotional and psychological aspects of the toy/activity

- Is play with the toy structured or unstructured?

- How much creativity and expression are required/allowed/facilitated?

- What motivates the child to engage with the toy?

- How much interaction, cooperation, sharing, turn-taking, conversation are involved? Does the toy/activity involve competition?

- How much choice is allowed?

- Does play with the toy provide a sense of control, competence, achievement?

- How challenging is the toy and how much opportunity is there for success?

  ☞ It is important that the toy/activity provides 'just the right amount of challenge' for the child.

  ☞ It is important that the child has a balance between high-tech and low-tech toys, as they require different levels of the above-mentioned requirements, such as hand manipulation, hands-on creativity.

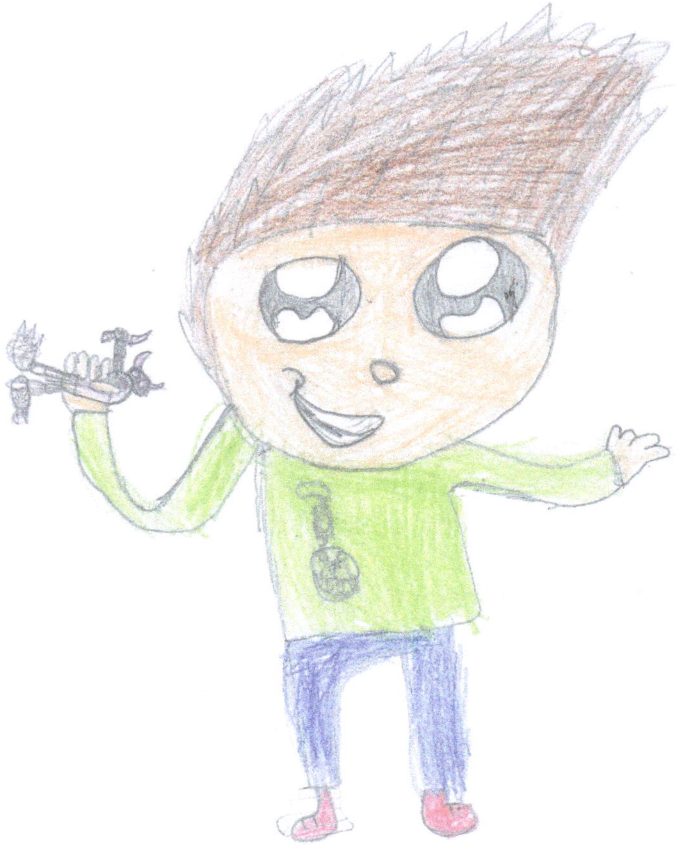

Wences, 8 years old, Spain

Toy or game adaptation

A child with disabilities might not be able to actively access, explore and take control of the toys and play materials. The toys and play promoted by the toys might not be suitable to his or her abilities.

Universal Design principles applied to toys may not completely eliminate the need for specific adaptations of toys. There are some commercially available adapted toys. Usually these are battery-operated toys in which it is possible to connect an external single switch to activate the toy, thus enabling children with motor impairments to use them. However, adapted toys are often expensive. Although they are assistive technology devices and, as such, they are eligible for public funding, many times in practice it is not easy to get funding when funds are scarce and allocation is primarily decided on base of medical considerations.

There are, however, many simple adaptations to assist the child in getting the most out of play. The purpose of these adaptations is usually related to stabilising, extending/building up, highlighting, attaching, confining and/or simplifying the toys/games.

Stabilising

Often toys that stay 'in one place' can be easier to use. Materials such as Velcro® fasteners, special grip rubber, or magnetic tape may assist play by securing a toy within the child's reach or vision.

Extending / Building Up

Materials like playdough lolly sticks or sponge rollers are used to build up certain access features. They help children press buttons or keys that are too small, or make markers and puzzle pieces easier to hold.

Highlighting Materials

Coloured Velcro® tape, Wikki Stix®, coloured masking tape, etc., are materials that can be used to highlight/enhance certain areas on toys, making them easier to locate. They help to simplify toy design and facilitate independent play by children.

Attaching

Materials such as snaps on fabric tape, elastic straps, or coloured Velcro® straps are used to bring items closer to the child, making reaching, grasping and playing less demanding.

Confining

Sometimes items are needed to create play areas that confine several toys. Materials such as hula hoops, box tops or planter bases, can prevent a toy from moving too far away from a child (out of the child's reach or vision). These items create boundaries to help a child control his immediate play environment. Their use may particularly benefit children with visual or physical impairments.

Simplifying

Try simplifying how play materials are presented to your child. Limiting the number of toy choices and pieces may make play easier. For example, by removing distractions from the play area before play begins. Select 1–2 toys at a time and place them on a contrasting colour surface.

Interfacing

Technological toys may be difficult to operate and proper interfaces may substitute the original ones: larger operating buttons, properly shaped handles, proper support providing stability, vocal commands instead of gestures or gestures instead of vocal interaction. Since, in some situations, the user can produce liquid secretions and technological tools may suffer from being wet, they could be protected (e.g. a joystick could be inserted in a plastic bag that could guarantee the good operability of the toy).

When a child is unable to play and use the provided toys, **an occupational therapist can help you:**

- Select toys or games that fit well both the child's interests, needs, abilities, and the family priorities and demands.

- Identify and recommend, for all age groups, accessible and safe toys and games that can challenge the child.

- Adapt or modify the child's toys and games, in order to support his/her participation and pleasure in play.

- Advise ways of using toys and games while considering the child, home or school routines and habits, and balance of play and work.

- Collaborate with families and educators to create opportunities that encourage the child to play with toys, promoting a sense of wellbeing.

When the required modifications may seem difficult to identify, design and implement, **an engineer or technician can help you:**

- Modify existing toys to match the player's needs and preferences and make it possible to play with a toy that would otherwise be hard to use.

- Add a dimension to animate the toy so that it can express signals that can be perceived by the player: movements, sounds, and lights. The player can explicitly decide to activate the mechanism. This makes it possible to create a cause-effect relationship that could be used both as a stimulus to induce interest and engagement, and as a reward for well-performed interactive actions.

- Program or re-program the toy to adapt it to the child's abilities, for example, modifications of the toy's actions and changes over time of the toy behaviour to keep the child engaged in the play.

Case study:

Simple ways for adapting a toy and enabling independent play with an age-appropriate toy - Story of Mark told by his occupational therapist

Mark was 3 years old when I first met him. He was diagnosed with severe cerebral palsy. Mark had a pronounced motor limitation; he was a very verbal and interactive child. He insisted on trying the same activities that his typically developing twin brother played with. He used his right hand (that had very limited movement) for stabilising the toys and his left hand for handling the toys themselves as best he could.

At that time, the favourite toy among Mark's peers was a bubble gun: a plastic toy gun that produced bubbles when the trigger was pressed. This commercial toy was unsuitable to Mark because it needed to be held with two hands: the soap container with one hand and the 'wand' with the other hand. It also needed to be stabilised to dip it in the soap solution. It needed fine oral-motor movements to blow air at the wand. Blowing virtual bubbles via a computer program or iPad was not an option for Mark; he insisted on using a 'real' bubble gun.

The solution we found for Mark to enable independent and group play using the bubble gun was adapting the gun for switch use. This meant creating a 'switch adapted toy', i.e. a toy that can be controlled by an external switch thus becoming accessible to all children. This provides a way for the child to make the toy go 'all by itself'. This possibility provides the means to self-generated, active engagement, as the ability to exert control becomes possible. It promotes a proactive attitude of 'I can do it!' leading to increased initiation attempts and empowerment. Using switches with toys develops play skills that include turning them on and off, moving them for social and communicative purposes, and making choices to indicate preferences, not to mention just having fun!

All one needs is a battery switch adaptor, which you can make or buy; you can also reach your Occupational Therapist to help you make one. You then can attach it to any simple battery operated toy of your preference and connect a switch to operate it, as in this example:

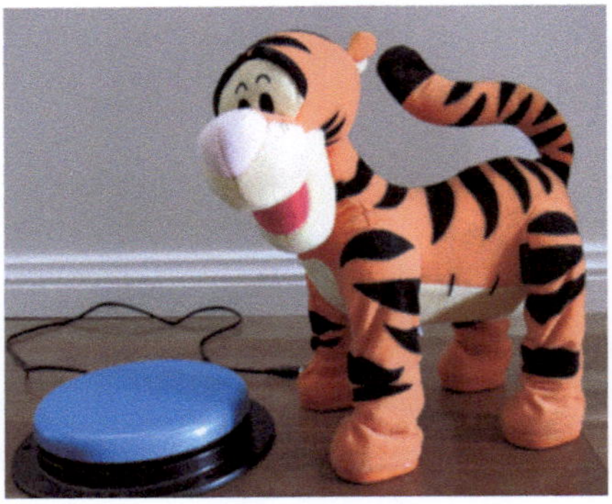

Switch-adapted Tiger

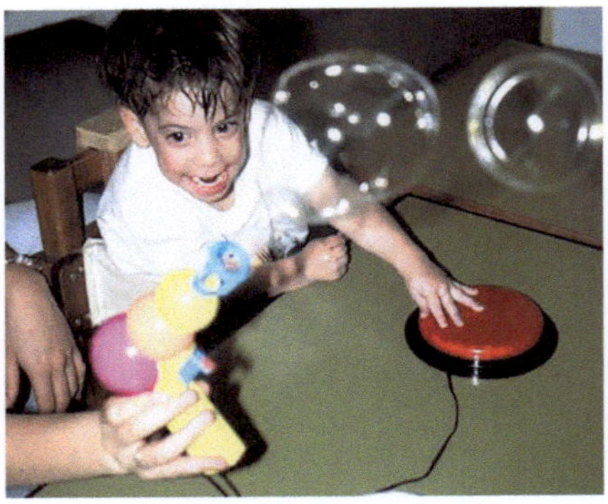

Mark - I can do it by myself !!!

It was Mark's choice to play with the bubble gun and therefore that is the toy we adapted. Mark used his left hand to press the switch that was connected with a battery switch adaptor to the bubble gun, thus enabling him to produce as many bubbles as he wanted and when he wanted! In this particular picture, an adult is holding the toy gun, but it could also have been attached to the table using a variety of kinds of support.

Playing with toys

Using mainstream toys with children with disabilities will be easier if they are displayed within a 'play framework'. This framework helps a child play freely, for fun, in confidence and control, and helps parents or caregivers become play mediators.

It comprises several elements:

1 – **An area dedicated to play freely** that the child knows is his/her special playspace. This area provides a feeling of control and emotional safety. It can be any suitable place where toys can be stored and spread out. Classrooms or rehabilitation rooms are usually unsuitable spaces for free play.

2 – **Several separated playspaces**, organized according to the toys' categories. For example, one for sensory-motor toys, a second for dolls and symbolic/pretend play, another for construction games and a fourth for rule play games.

3 – **Well-chosen challenging toys and games**, displayed within playspaces, one by one and not in a jumble, so that the child can easily understand his/her play environment.

4 – **Adults as play mediators** and belonging to the play framework, where they encourage the child to access and explore the toys by him/herself, and adapt their behaviours so that the child can lead the play. For example, adults may start the play session with the child rediscovering some of the toys that have already been used. Then, gradually introduce different toys that allow the child to recombine mastered skills in new play situations. Please refer to Chapter 5 for more details on the adult's role in play contexts.

5 – **Clearly defined rules** for use of the playspaces and toys, so that the child can adapt his/her actions and behaviours: for example, toys must not be thrown away.

Conclusion

- Toys and games are objects that support children's play.
- There are toys and games for different categories/types of play.
- They should be chosen according to the players' capacities and interests and the social and physical context of play.
- Toys and games with Universal Design features are more likely to be used successfully by children with disabilities.
- When children cannot access and use toys and games, there still are many simple adaptations and possibilities to frame the play in order to assist the child in getting the most out of the play experience.

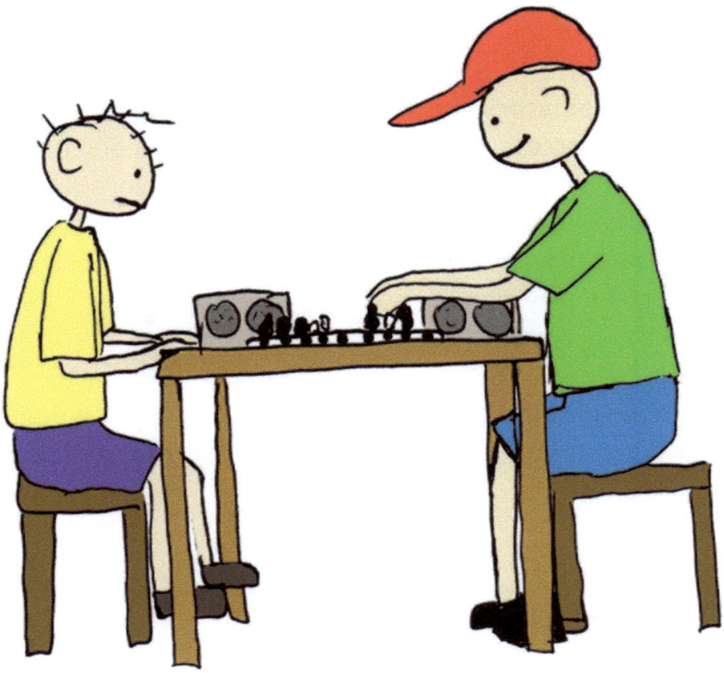

Mihaela, 16 years old, Croatia

8

Which digital games are appropriate for our children?

Agnieszka Landowska

The advancement of computer science plays a vital role in the modern society, with a possible positive impact in the quality of life of diverse groups of people, including children with disabilities. Nowadays, there is a significant number of digital games designed specifically to meet special needs of children. In addition, a large percentage of all the available digital games is designed to be also accessible to people with various types of impairments.

If the ocean of digital games is too intimidating for you to explore, this chapter provides a guided excursion helping you to understand how to support your child with disabilities in the use of digital games for play purposes. Digital games that run on computers, tablets or smart phones are considered; digital games for video game consoles are outside the scope of this chapter.

Does your child want to use a computer, a tablet or a smart phone?

Most children do. Most of them actually love to. As children frequently observe adults playing or working with computers, tablets and smart phones, they find the interaction with electronic devices highly attractive and satisfying. In fact, if your child is not interested in computers, tablets and smart phones, you should probably consider encouraging him/her towards using them. These electronic devices may play the role of a window to the outside world, being a medium for inclusiveness, social life, work and entertainment throughout the entire life of your child.

Are digital games appropriate for children?

The appropriateness of digital games depends on the child's age, skills and interests, and the games themselves. Carefully selected games may support a child's play experience. However, it is quite important to emphasise that the use of electronic devices such as computers, tablets and smart phones by a child, with or without disabilities, should be to some extent controlled or assisted by adults. The latter should not allow, for example, a child to sit and play on a computer for hours. Instead, the adult should encourage more physically and socially demanding play activities, such as those that require physical exercise and/or interaction between playmates. The younger a child is, the shorter the time allowed for digital games should be.

How to create a proper environment for a child to play with digital games

A proper environment is necessary to make the use of digital games easy, safe and beneficial for your child. There are six steps to follow:

Step 1. Choosing the proper device.

There is a variety of devices that can be used to run digital games, including smart phones, tablets, notebooks and desktop computers. Usually, for children a tablet is preferable over a notebook or a desktop computer, mainly due transportability and to the intuitiveness of using a finger to control the device instead of a pointing system like a mouse or trackpad. In fact, children with intellectual impairments, dyspraxia or with autism spectrum disorders may have difficulties in understanding the connection between mouse and cursor movements. Tablets come in different sizes. For small (kindergarten) children, a 7" device is a good option, given that it is easy to transport and manipulate. When a child has motor or visual impairments, bigger is better. There are large tablets in the market and it is also possible to opt for a notebook or even a desktop computer with touch screens. You lose in transportability, but a bigger screen will allow your child independent access to the device. Remember that a tablet can be easily dropped from the hands of a child. There are several child friendly cases available in the market. These are fun and offer extra-protection.

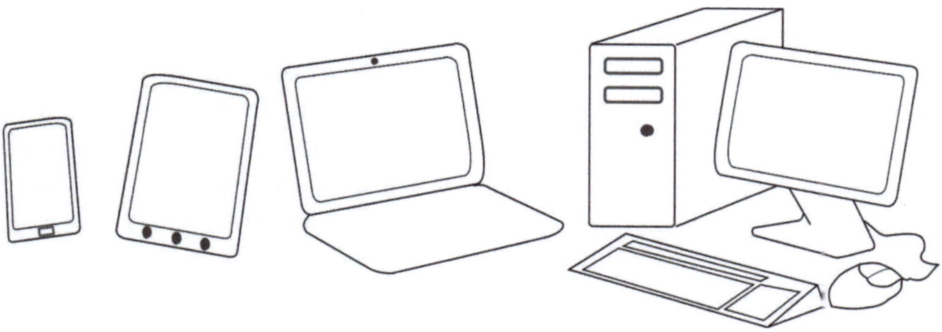

A choice of devices: smart phones, tablets, notebooks, desktop computers

Another aspect to take into account is the device operating system. Most common are Android, iOS (from Apple) and Windows. Windows devices are losing popularity and fewer applications are available for them; Android devices are usually cheaper than iOS (Apple) devices. Avoid buying devices with proprietary operating systems – there will be much less applications available for them. Remember also that operating systems are incompatible with each other, meaning that an application for an operating system does not run in a device with another operating system. Therefore, if you already have a device, it might be preferable to keep with your previous choice of operating system.

Step 2. Choosing proper digital games.

There are so many digital games that a person can easily feel overwhelmed without knowing which ones are appropriate or not. You should always keep in mind that play is all about your child having fun. You should thus focus on the interests and preferences of your child and look for a game that will motivate him/her to play (e.g. if your child is fond of Mickey Mouse, look for games where he appears). In order to assess a particular game, it is worth considering the following characteristics:

- Age appropriateness – Games are designed for specific age groups, sometimes being possible to adjust them for different targets. When considering age appropriateness, take into consideration not only the chronological age, but also developmental age. Note that it is not appropriate to propose a very difficult game for a child but it is equally not appropriate to propose a too simple one. Children like to be challenged when playing. The secret is to find the right amount of challenge.

- Motor skills required – A digital game always requires some interaction with the child. It is crucial to understand what are the motor skills required by the game and, if there is a gap between those and the child's skills, evaluate if it can be bridged adapting the game or using assistive technology. Some games provide accessibility options such as adjustable size of the control buttons, or are switch compatible (meaning they can be controlled through a single switch).

- Vision skills required – Most of the games are designed for sighted people. There are, however, games designed for people with low vision or even blind. These use auditory cues that enable a child with vision impairments to master them. Haptic feedback is also possible since most smart phones and tables are able to vibrate.

- Language requirements – Most games require some level of language understanding (both for understanding instructions and for playing). Keep in mind that your child should be able to play autonomously. Although you can provide some initial support, overcoming possible difficulties in understanding the game instructions, your child should be able to play by him/herself after a while.

Below you can find more information on what to look for when assessing digital games for different groups of children.

Step 3. Improving accessibility of the device, if needed.

For a child with disabilities it may be challenging to access a computer or a tablet. There are several assistive products, both hardware and software, that can assist the child, including

- Alternative input devices, such as switches, adapted mice, joysticks or keyboards, voice control software;

- Headphones, screen magnifiers (there are hardware options, attachable to a screen, and also software options that interface with a computer's graphical output to present enlarged screen content);

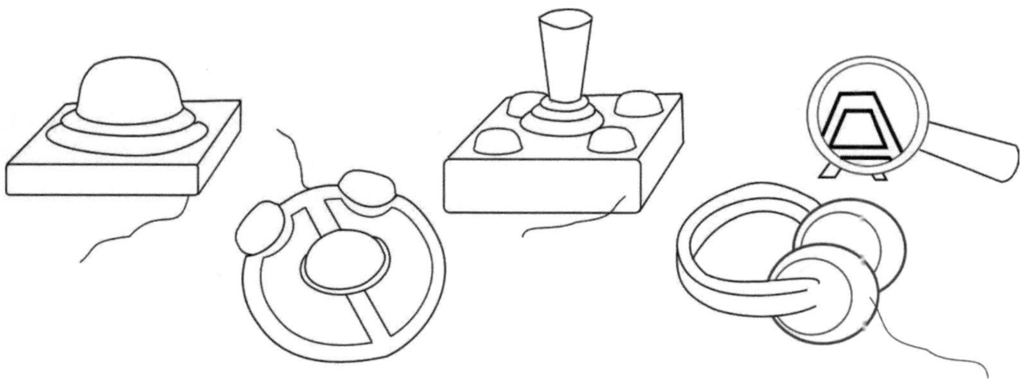

Examples of assistive products that may facilitate the access to a computer: single switches, adapted mice and joysticks, headphones, magnifiers

- Screen readers (software that uses speech synthesis to read aloud the information on a display).

Make sure you check the Accessibility Options of your device's operating system. They will allow you to adjust sound volume; screen brightness, contrast, and colour scheme; voice control and screen reading; font size; and mouse speed, among other options. It might be also worth to consider adapting the way to turn on and off the device such that the child becomes independent in its use.

Please refer to Chapter 6 for more details on Assistive Technology that may support your child in accessing an electronic device.

Step 4. Organising the environment.

Use of computers and tablets should be safe, for both your child and the device. Please consider the following:

- Location of the device – Tablets and computers are usually safe on a desk or table. You can use special holders, non-slip mat or even adhesive tape to fix the device to the desk or table. If sitting at a desk is not an option for your child, you may consider putting the device on the floor and have the child sitting or lying on the floor. Make sure the child can comfortably see the display by adjusting the position of it with respect to the child (placing the display such that ¼ of the screen is above eye-level is a good starting rule of thumb) and by paying attention to light sources and screen tilting to reduce glare.

- Device setup – Be sure to have in advance everything ready for the child to play, including any assistive products that might be needed to support the child. Play should be seen by the child as a moment for fun and recreational pleasure, not as a long process of setting up everything culminating in using a game when he/she is no longer in the mood.

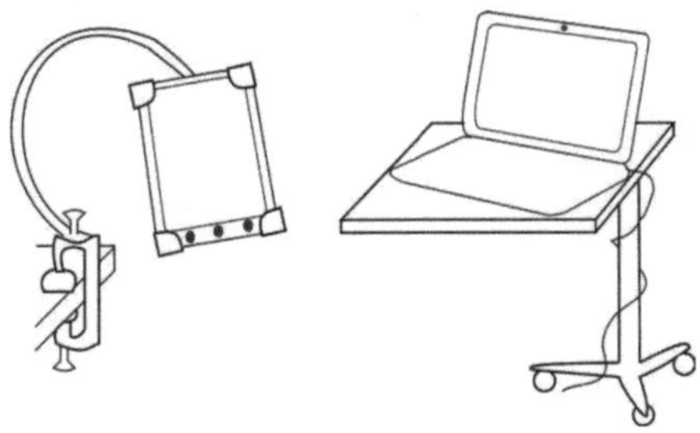

Different options to set up electronic devices

- Child's comfort – Make sure that the child body position is appropriate (stable, safe and comfortable), feet flat on the floor or on a footrest, especially when you plan a longer interaction session (be warned that it usually takes longer than expected).

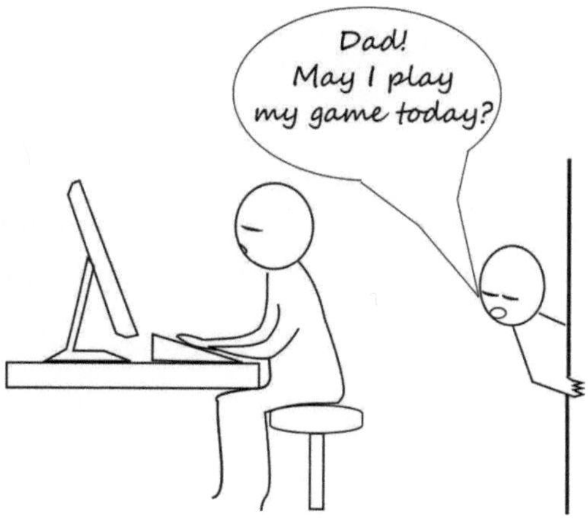

Step 5. Playing yourself first.

When considering a digital game, download and install it (most of them have trial versions) and play yourself first. Evaluate whether it is appropriate and enjoyable from the child's perspective. Explore the game settings. In particular, look for options for: sound volume, speed, different graphics and/or content, and accessibility features. Remember to play the game as your child will (e.g. using the same assistive product, if he/she will be using one).

Step 6. Assisting and adapting.

Allow your child enough time to explore and try the game. Provide support when needed, but only when needed. Please refer to Chapter 5 for more details on the adult role when supporting children's play. Respect your child preferences and be flexible - a child might not enjoy every game you have chosen. Make the necessary adaptations to the environment, if needed. Sometimes adding adhesive tape here and there makes a huge difference. Consider also setting some

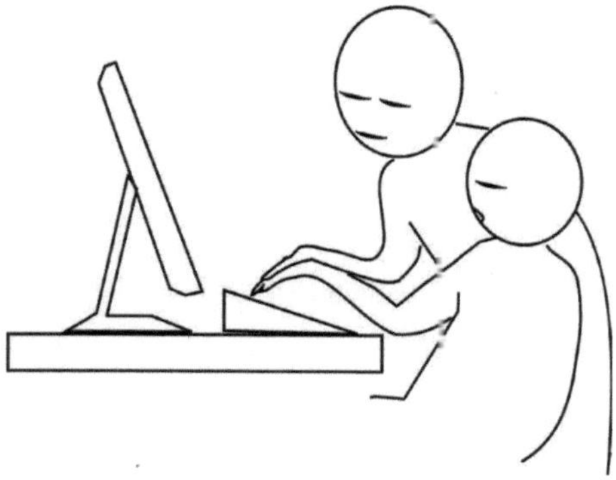

Hand-on-hand assistance

rules on the use of digital games (e.g. define time limits, name inappropriate behaviours). With older children using the Internet, social media or YouTube videos, consider setting parental control on the device.

Digital games for children with visual impairments

Visual impairments are quite diverse. Colour vision impairment usually is not very limitative when using digital games. Adjusting contrast and colours, in the game itself or at the operating system level, may provide the necessary adaptation for these users.

When choosing a digital game for a child with mild to medium visual impairments consider the following issues:

- Background – Background should be plain or there should be the possibility of choosing a plain background. The more details or patterns in the background, the less visible are the buttons and other controls on the foreground.

- Foreground – Foreground should also be as simple as possible, showing only the relevant visual information. Ideally, it should be possible to adjust the size of buttons and other controls making them as big as twice an adult fingertip.

- Background/foreground contrast – Contrast between background and foreground should be high in both colour and brightness. The game should provide options to change contrast.

- Auditory feedback and alternative text – Controls and different actions should provide auditory feedback. Images and videos should have text descriptions providing access to non-text information to screen reader users.

- Screen-reader compatibility – Digital games should be compatible with screen readers to increase their accessibility for children with vision impairments.

- Consistency throughout the game – Position of the different game controls and their relative position should not change from screen to screen.

For children with very low vision or blind you need to consider a bigger device and the use of screen readers and voice control software. As mentioned above, digital games for blind children should rely on auditory and haptic feedback only.

Digital games for children with motor impairments

For children that will be interacting with the device using their hands, despite their motor impairments, the following should be considered:

- Required gestures – Using a device with a touch screen requires the ability to perform several gestures:

  ☞ Single finger gestures – Tap and double tap, tap and hold (touch and hold position), swipe (moving a finger on the screen), flick (fast swipe), drag-and-drop (tap and swipe).

  ☞ Two fingers gestures: pinch inwards and outwards, rotate (spin the fingers in a circle).

  Gestures required for using a digital game should be assessed in comparison to the child's skills. Alternative control methods should be available if the child is not able to perform the required gestures.

- Error tolerance – Evaluate the game behaviour upon involuntary touches on the screen, possibly with several fingers simultaneously. Is the action reversible?

- Adjustable controls size – Buttons and other on-screen controls should be big enough (at least one adult fingertip) and have enough space between them to facilitate use for children with fine motor impairments.

For children unable to use their hands to directly access the device or unable to use a standard keyboard or mouse, alternative input devices must be sought. Voice control is an option for those children that are able to clearly articulate words. Eye-tracking systems, where the cursor is controlled through eyeball movements, are another alternative. Single switches require minimum motor skills and often are the only usable input device for children with severe motor impairments. However, games should be compatible with switch control and that is usually only possible for very simple games with a linear flow. Note that it takes time to master an alternative input device and that often these are less effective than traditional input devices. Try it yourself!

Digital games for children with hearing impairments

Digital games are mostly visual mediums, therefore they are usually accessible to children with hearing impairments. In any case, you should consider the following when selecting a digital game for a child with hearing impairments:

- Sound dependency – Although most digital games are visual, there are some which rely heavily on sounds (e.g. games featuring the 'voices' of animals). If you are considering such a game, you should verify if your child hearing skills enable him/her to take pleasure from the game. In some games, auditory instructions and/or feedback are provided (e.g. cheering sound upon completing a task). There should be also a visual feedback (e.g. showing a cheering image in complement to the sound).

- Background sound – Digital games are usually associated with background melodies or sounds that are not essential for playing them. These may make it harder for children with mild/medium hearing impairments to concentrate on the relevant sounds (e.g. spoken instructions) and thus it should be possible to turn them off.

- Sound volume control – It should be possible to control the game sound volume.

Digital games for children with autism spectrum disorders

Children with autism spectrum disorders are usually fond of electronic devices. This preference is typically attributed to predictability and repetitiveness of the interaction with the devices. Since autism is a spectrum disorder, there is a wide variation in the skills of children with this diagnosis. The following aspects may or may not be worth considering for your particular child when assessing a digital game:

- Sound – If a child is sensitive to sound, it should be possible to control the game sound volume. You may also consider the use of headphones that contribute to isolate the child from the outside world and concentrate on the game.

- Consistency throughout the game – Position of the different game controls and their relative position should not change from screen to screen. Same actions should always lead to the same effects.

- Adjustable content – Some children with autism spectrum disorders may have problems in recognizing objects in unfamiliar scenarios or in interpreting symbolic representations (e.g. smiley icon as a representation of joy). Those would benefit from a customizable game where, for example, it is possible to use own pictures.

- Robustness – Some children with autism spectrum disorders like to explore digital games by randomly and quickly tapping on the screen, sometimes leading them to the game settings page or somewhere else outside the usual game flow. There should always be a clear way of returning to a familiar game screen.

Digital games for children with intellectual disabilities

Intellectual disabilities are quite diverse. However, there are some common issues that should be considered:

- Plain scenarios – Simple game scenarios, without any unnecessary content, may facilitate the use of the game.

- Simple and intuitive interaction – The way to interact with the digital game should be clear, easy to remember, including the way to start it (e.g. games where there is a number of options that need to be chosen before starting to play should be avoided). The game should be error-proof or at least it should be easy to recover from errors (e.g. it should be possible and easy to reverse an action).

- Game flow – Digital games with a linear and static flow, rather than having multiple branches that require user decisions or being time varying, are preferable. If decisions are needed, no more than two options should be offered to the user.

- Adjustable difficulty – Since a child does not enjoy a challenge beyond his/her abilities, digital games should feature different levels of difficulty. Although this is often the case, progression between levels is usually assumed to be very fast. It should be possible for the user to choose the difficulty level, instead of forcing an automatic progression when one level is completed.

Conclusion

With all the electronic devices and digital games available today, there are surely at least a few digital games that are accessible to your child and that your child will enjoy playing with. Entertainment is a state somewhere between frustration and boredom. When choosing a digital game one needs to consider the child abilities and the skills required by the game so the child can enjoy it. Good games are those that provide just the right amount of challenge. Adults should always take into consideration the children's perspectives and preferences. Many times children enjoy games that are meaningless to adults. Remember that play is about recreational pleasure and enjoyment!

9

Which playspaces are appropriate for our children?

Helen Lynch[3]

Play and playspaces

As we have seen in earlier chapters, play is fundamental to how the child engages in the world. Enabling play requires a combination of factors; but the most playful events are usually a result of having a strong match between the child's play needs, and the **just-right challenge** in the social and physical environment. These environments are often called playspaces: **playspace** is a term applied to any place where a child plays, such as parks, greens, and yards, and is not limited to a purpose-built playground.

Therefore, before thinking about spaces for play, it is important to think about your child, your family, and your play needs. While play is something you know about as a carer or parent, you may not be aware that it is highly influenced by you, your family, your culture as well as your child's play needs and preferences.

In relation to your child, think about:

- How does s/he like to play?
- What are his/her play preferences?
- Where does s/he like to play?

3 With thanks to Dr Maria Prellwitz and Dr Christina Schulze for their input on this text.

- Where do his/her friends like to play?
- Are there local places they go?
- What are the main challenges for play for your child?
- In the ideal world, what would enable your child to play?

In relation to you, your family, your culture, and context, think about:

- What do you like to play, what is important to you and your family?
- What kind of spaces do you have available for play, for the whole family or just for the child?
- Where do you like to go as a family to play?
- What are the main challenges for you and your family for play?
- In the ideal world, what would be your play solution?

For example, for some families playing together is very important, while for others the adults like to provide play opportunities for their children but prefer to engage in more adult-like sport activities. Knowing your play style as a family is an important place to start. You and your child are the experts in knowing what is important for play in your family!

Playspaces

So how can we find playspaces that have the **just-right challenge** for your child? Once you have thought about what is important to you and your family, next, we need to understand the core characteristics of playspaces, and explore **which spaces are appropriate for our children for play.**

Play can happen anywhere: at the kitchen table, in the sitting room, out the back garden, in front of the home, in the car, along the footpath, at school or in a local town park playground. We know from research that children use many places for play in different counties, including derelict sites, waterfronts, parking lots. These examples show that sometimes play takes place in public settings, or designated play settings, but play also happens in unexpected places. The important thing children say about these places, is that they are fun (high in **play value**), and they are places to gather and meet friends. **Play value** means that there are play opportunities available that the children can access and use, and wish to use. These opportunities often include loose parts such as sticks, sand or water: they do not always involve purchased toys.

Therefore, playspaces are any place a child uses for play. For your child, and for your family, think of a favourite playspace that offers high play value, and consider:

- What environmental features makes this playspace successful? Space? Safety hazards? Accessibility? Variety of stimulation?

- How can your child play successfully in this playspace?

- If there are some parts of this playspace that do not work so well, can play be enabled with adaptation to the environment, or by providing physical help?

This picture shows an example of a playspace that has been designed to maximise accessibility for a range of different children, with different abilities and play needs by designing accessible routes and surfaces:

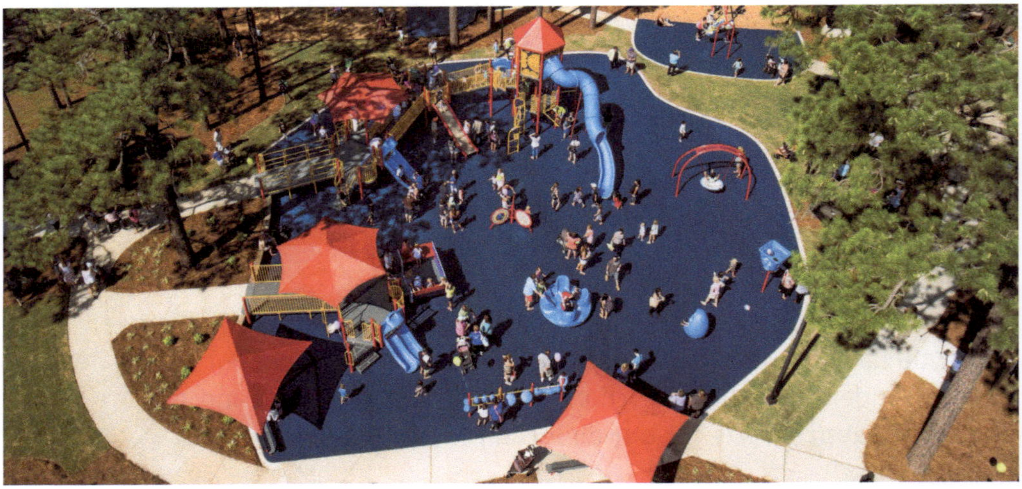

Source: PlayCore®

How the physical environment supports play: matching the child needs with the design of the built environment in accessing play opportunities

It is likely that you have many ideas about why some playspaces work well for your family and your child, and other playspaces do not. It maybe that you can see times when your child's disability is affecting his/her play opportunities. This can be due to difficulties in motor, sensory, cognitive, social, or emotional skills and abilities. However, it can also be attributed to the design of the environment (including toys or playspaces). For example, a child with visual impairments may not enjoy visits to a typical playground, but if the playground is designed with visual features to maximise accessibility, then this can make a significant difference. Similarly, if playground components are designed with multiple users in mind, everyone can play together. Figure below shows how having a carefully designed play component promotes social play

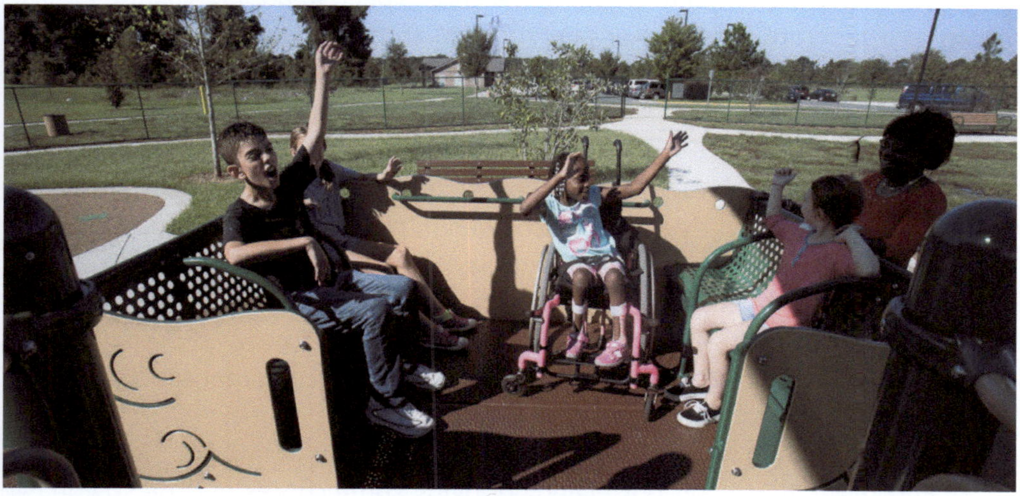

Source: PlayCore®

This example introduces the idea of finding the **just-right environment**: a just-right environment is one that has the best match between the child's play needs, the family/social needs and the opportunities in the physical environment.

Where is the just-right environment at home?

Children with disabilities spend more time at home than children without disabilities and so potentially play happens more frequently at home than elsewhere. Play at home involves family and friends, when playdates are organised for the child. The physical space available to the child and the characteristics of the environment and the availability of play materials and partners influence children's participation in play. It is therefore important that parents are well informed and aware of how to make home environment accessible for play. From what we know in research, children report that their homes are the most usable playspaces, which shows that parents are most effective at adapting the home space according to their child's needs, compared to school and community settings.

Although there may be many play preferences for home-based play, studies have shown that typical play choices include watching TV, and playing computer games for children with different disabilities in Ireland, Canada, and Sweden. Enabling play so that friends can play together is a core aspect. In addition, some families organise a separate play area or play room to support play. As we noted earlier, this is often linked with your family preferences or your cultural perspective on how places in the home are used.

However, many children prefer to be near other family members and so, providing nearby playspaces might be more successful in the home. For example, for children who are at the exploratory stage of play:

- Have play activities in the kitchen for when adults need to prepare meals (e.g. have a bottom drawer or cupboard shelf with kitchen utensils for the child to explore and play alongside while you cook);

- Encourage more outdoor play by bringing some chores outside so you can work alongside your child if they are playing in sand trays or exploring in the garden.

Where is the just-right environment outdoors?

Play in Communities

There are many challenges in finding outdoor play solutions for children in many countries, including children with disabilities. With an increase in city living and urbanisation, families are challenged to find welcoming community playspaces. This includes families of children with disabilities. For example, in studies of playgrounds, researchers have found that many playgrounds are not designed to be accessible, or if they are, the play value or challenge is missing.

However, families in urban settings have also been exploring new ways to provide play in their communities. One example is the Playing Out initiative in the UK. This is a community strengths-based approach to enabling play, where families plan to gather on a regular basis and enable play on their street. Permission is gained from the Municipality to temporarily close the street where the community lives (e.g. once a week for two hours). The community members gather on the street to support their children to play together; no traffic is allowed through the street during this time. See link in Chapter 11 to Child-in-the-City for more information.

In other contexts, families of children with Autism Spectrum Disorders (ASD) have worked on solutions to designing just-right environments that are autism-friendly. For example, one initiative that has been growing in popularity recently, is to have a 'disability-friendly' time in a supermarket for shopping. During this allotted time, the noise levels are reduced to accommodate children with ASD who have sensory sensitivities. In other research studies, parents have suggested that something similar needs to be done for playgrounds: to ask the local playground manager to hold special times each week that are 'disability-friendly'. The goal here is to work towards inclusion, and reduce segregation and stigma, so that families of children with special needs can go to the playground and not be anxious about feeling unwelcome. Their suggestion shows that sometimes small steps are needed to work towards inclusion in a community. By developing initiatives such as in the Playing Out programme or by having special times in a public setting, communities can change and play can be enabled. See Chapter 11 for some links.

Play in Schools

As schools are places where children spend a significant amount of time, they provide an important source of play opportunity also for children with impairments. However, in many countries, families and educators have reported increasing pressures from the school curriculum to reduce time spent in free play. Furthermore, in some countries such as Ireland, outdoor play areas in schools are places to run about, with no play equipment to foster other forms of play.

In recent years, it is exciting to see how play experts have responded to these problems, for example:

1. Schools are being targeted now as sites for promoting physical activity play (see Chapter 11 for examples from Australia and the USA). In the USA study, the researchers adapted the physical, built environment to increase play activity. These adaptations included: having garden areas, providing wheeled toy pathways, providing natural elements such as logs, rocks and shrubs. Similarly, in the Australian study, Bundy and colleagues introduced 'loose materials' which is the term for objects with no apparent play value, such as ropes, empty boxes, and wood. Her study has shown how play can be enabled using such materials for all children in a cost-effective way.

2. This renewed focus on play and the schoolyard has led to a new movement called **schoolyard greening**, which refers to changes made to school environments to restore natural elements within them. Schoolyard greening is taking place in North America, Australia, the UK and Northern Europe based on the strong evidence that green school yards encourage more active play, promote positive behaviour as well as augment play and learning. Thus, schools provide a rich environment in which children can engage with nature and the outdoors.

However, there are still no clear, universally accepted guidelines on how to provide accessible playgrounds in schools and public settings (see Chapter 3, on play policy and barriers). The next section looks at Universal Design as the way forward in finding a solution for communities everywhere.

Playspaces: Universal Design, usability and accessibility

With some thought and careful planning, community playspaces can be designed for maximum play value, to provide the **just-right challenge** for children of all abilities. Universal Design is the approach that can enable such design. Universal Design (UD) is about making products usable for people of all abilities. When a place is universally designed, it is both accessible **and** usable. Accessible means that the space is a place where you and your child can get to: for example, to get to the local play park or playground. Accessible environments are usually guided by minimum standards set out in legislation in each country. Universal Design goes beyond minimum standards for accessibility however: it also includes usability.

Usability means that once you get there, you can use the play opportunities that are there: for example, to climb the slide or use the swing.

Applying UD to playground design is quite new, and has not yet been researched in any great detail; however, it provides us with some important considerations and guides us in designing just-right environments for play.

Good playground design for accessibility and usability considers varied needs of the broadest range of users possible. For example:

1. For families with physical impairments

- Providing a firm pathway to the playground to ensure accessibility.

- Avoiding the use of sand or loose wood chippings around play components (swings, slides, climbing frames) so that people with wheelchairs can make their way about easily.

2. For families with visual impairments

- Providing clear information that outlines the route in playground so that people with limited sight can visualise the route through the space (e.g. through using maps/braille).

- Use of colour to denote edges of pathways or play components.

3. For families with social-emotional impairments

- Providing places for solitary play in the playspace for a child who gets easily overwhelmed and who may need a short time away from others during play activity.

4. For families with intellectual disabilities

- Providing a clear layout of the playspace so that it is easy to follow and use independently.

- Having equipment that is self- explanatory in how it is to be used (intuitive).

PlayCore® is one organisation in the United States that has developed tools to help designers and municipalities to design playgrounds from a UD perspective. Seven principles of UD have been identified:

1. Equitable Use: Be Fair!
2. Flexibility in Use: Be Included!
3. Simple and Intuitive: Be Smart!
4. Perceptible Information: Be Independent!
5. Tolerance for Error: Be Safe!
6. Low Physical Effort: Be Active!
7. Size and Space for Approach: Be Comfortable!

However, it is also important to figure out how to design playgrounds that are fun, that have a high play value. Universal Design is an important way for considering how accessible and usable a place is for a **person**. But we need to go beyond focusing on the person and make sure we also focus on what happens there: **play**. This is currently the focus of a number of projects in Europe, and also among researchers from the International Play Association – links to some examples are provided in Chapter 11.

Universal Design and the just-right environment: exploring solutions

Based on our knowledge of play, every playground has some play components (i.e. swings, climbing frames, slides) that **are not** usable by all children. Playgrounds need to provide challenge and have some play challenges that are too difficult for some children or too easy for others. This is because playgrounds need to cater for different play skills and abilities. It is therefore important to note that playgrounds cannot be fully accessible: if this was the case, the play value may be missing.

In the Netherlands, there is an interesting example of how one project has developed to address this issue. Play workers have set up an organisation to assess the play value of local playgrounds, using the experts (children!) to carry out the assessment. A national programme has been put in place aiming:

- For every playground to be 100% welcome,
- With 70% accessibility,
- With 50% usability.

This message clearly establishes the need to understand that for every child, playgrounds cannot be 100% accessible, otherwise there may not be any challenge and the playspace may inadvertently be boring for the child!

Development of an Audit tool for playground assessment

For a Universal Design project in Ireland, a Playground Audit tool was developed to help assess playspaces. The Audit tool gathers together questions to consider: accessibility, usability, natural elements for play, built environment for play, and play preferences.

The current version of this tool can be found in the Appendix to this book. It is currently being used in research to see if it can help designers, landscape architects, playground workers, to plan for public playgrounds that are **Universally Designed for People and Play**.

Conclusion

- Play can happen anywhere and in any place, but the most valuable play happens when there is a **JUST-RIGHT CHALLENGE** in the physical and social environment.

- Playspaces can be structured or unstructured. Plan to develop play opportunities where your child likes to play. This can be near you at home or with friends in the street. By careful planning and using your insight of your child's needs and what is available to you, you will be able to figure out which places are appropriate for our children: the **JUST-RIGHT ENVIRONMENTS**.

- When playspaces are structured, they need to be designed with Universal Design in mind, i.e. designed for accessibility and usability.

- However, playgrounds should not be designed to be 100% accessible and usable, as this would mean that they may have limited play challenge and therefore reduced play value.

10

Take home messages

Pedro Encarnação, Sylvie Ray-Kaeser, Nicole Bianquin and Serenella Besio

Below you can find a list of key ideas about play for children with disabilities that we would like you to reflect on upon reading this book:

- 'Play is a range of voluntary, intrinsically motivated activities associated with recreational pleasure and enjoyment'.

- Traits of play include being a child-lead activity, freely chosen, with no other goals besides the fun of playing.

- Playful activities with educational or therapeutic goals, although being an invaluable means to engage children, are not play but play-like activities.

- Play for the sake of play supports all aspects of a child's development and well-being.

- Play is a right for all children enshrined in international conventions such as the United Nations Convention on the Rights of the Child or the United Nations Convention on the Rights of Persons with Disabilities.

- Disability does not lie solely in the person, it is the result of a complex interaction between a person, with his/her health condition, abilities and personal factors, and the environment, including the physical, social, cultural and institutional contexts. Disability is the outcome of a misfit between a person and an environment with barriers (or without proper facilitators), restricting individual's activities and participation.

- Children with disabilities have the same desire to play as any other children. Play is equally important for their development and well-being. Moreover, play is the natural way for them to interact with peers, thus fostering inclusion.

- Children with disabilities face many barriers to play, including

  - institutional barriers (the importance of play is recognized by all in theory, but there's a lack of active play promotion policies);

  - social-cultural barriers (play often occupies a secondary role when compared to educational or therapeutic activities, sometimes children with disabilities are ostracized of feel stigmatized); and

  - physical barriers (lack of accessible playspaces, toys, games).

- Direct observation is the best way of assessing children's play. There are several questionnaires and observation grids that can support play assessment. This assessment is instrumental in planning proper interventions such that a child can fully enjoy his/her right to play for the sake of play.

- Play can be learned and taught.

- Adults can guide and support children with disabilities to play. It is fundamental that adults keep in mind what is play ensuring that their interventions do not jeopardize the children's play experience. The metaphor of scaffolding is particularly illustrative: adults should provide the support that is needed but, once children acquire the skills needed to play, adults should step down and allow children to take full control of the play.

- Play often requires staying in a comfortable and functional position, moving around, manipulating objects, communicating, or using a computer or tablet. There is a vast number of assistive products that may reduce the gap between the requirements of the play and the children's abilities by providing support in the above general-purpose functional areas or by adapting the activity.

- The secret of keeping a child engaged in play is providing the just-right amount of challenge. Too much challenge leads to frustration; too little challenge leads to boredom.

- There are no toys, games, playspaces suitable for every child and family. Each child and each family is unique, with his or her own preferences and interests. There are, however, general principles that can help enabling play for everyone.

- Play is not an attribute of toys and games; play belongs to the players. Although toys and games are tools for play, children can play with whatever is available. They certainly don't need expensive toys in order to play.

- Toys and games should be accessible to the widest range of abilities possible; they should be designed in order to match the motor, sensory, perceptual, cognitive, socio-emotional and psychological skills of the broadest possible group of children (not too easy, not too complicated, the just-right amount of challenge).

- Children nowadays are usually attracted by electronic devices and digital games. Although there is the need of ensuring enough opportunities for more physically and socially demanding play activities, children should not be prohibited from playing with digital games as it will develop skills they will need to live in our digital world.

- It is not all about the toy and the game. Although play can happen anywhere, a dedicated space and time for play, with the right toys and (if needed) the right assistive products, the right playmates and the right play context can better enable the child to play.

- The play value of a space refers to the amount of play opportunities available that the children can access or use, and wish to use.

- A playground with high play value, that provides the just-right amount of challenge for every child, will have some components that are not usable by all children. A rule of thumb might be: a playground should be 100% welcoming, 70% accessible and 50% usable.

- Play in natural environments should also be accessible to children with disabilities.

- It will only be play if the child is in control and feels involved. Make sure to properly assess the particular preferences and interests of a child, and seek the child's opinion. The experts on play are the children!

- A new culture of play for all, especially for children with disabilities, is needed. Societies should internalize the invaluable importance of play for the sake of play and strive for policies that ensure that all children can enjoy their right to play.

11

Information resources on play for children with disabilities

Chapter 1 – What is play?

For more information on play definitions please refer to:

Bateson, G. (1956). *The Message "This Is Play".* Princeton, NJ, USA: Josia Macy Jr. Foundation.

Besio, S. (2017). The Need for Play for the Sake of Play. In S. Besio, D. Bulgarelli, & V. Stancheva-Popkostadinova (Eds.), *Play Development in Children with Disabilities* (pp. 9-52). Warsaw, Poland: De Gruyter Poland.

Besio, S. (2018). Supporting the Play for the Sake of Play in Children with Disabilities. *Today's Children Tomorrow's Parents*, 47-48, 7-17.

Bondioli, A. (2002). *Gioco e educazione* [Play and education]. Milano, Italy: Franco Angeli.

Bruner, J. S. (1986). *Actual Minds, Possible Worlds.* Cambridge, MA, USA: Harvard University Press.

Bulgarelli, D., & Bianquin, N. (2017). Conceptual Review of Play. In S. Besio, D. Bulgarelli, & V. Stancheva-Popkostadinova (Eds.), *Play Development in Children with Disabilities* (pp. 58-70). Warsaw, Poland: De Gruyter Poland.

Burghardt, G. (2005) *The Genesis of Animal Play. Testing the Limits.* Cambridge, MA, USA: The MIT Press.

Caillois, R. (1961). *Man, Play and Games.* Champaign, IL, USA: University of Illinois Press.

Dewey, J. (1944). *Democracy and Education.* New York, NY, USA: Macmillan.

Fénelon, F. (2000). *The Education of a Child from the Wisdom of Fénelon 1687.* Mount Norris, NY, USA: Lamplighter Publishing.

Fröbel, F. (2012). *The Education of Man.* New York, NY, USA: Dover Publications.

Garvey, C. (1990). *Play.* Cambridge, MA, USA: Harvard University Press.

Hewett, V. M. (2001). Examining the Reggio Emilia Approach to Early Childhood Education. *Early Childhood Education Journal*, 29(2), 95-100.

Locke, J. (1824). Some Thoughts Concerning Education. In J. Locke, *The works of John Locke in nine volumes (vol. 8)*. Retrieved from http://oll.libertyfund.org/titles/locke-the-works-vol-8-some-thoughts-concerning-education-posthumous-works-familiar-letters

Montessori, M. (1996). *The Secret of Childhood.* Asheville, NC, USA: Longmans, Green and Company.

Parten, M. B. (1932). Social participation among pre-school children. *Journal of Abnormal and Social Psychology*, 27, 243-269.

Piaget, J. (1962). *Play, Dreams and Imitation in Childhood*, New York, NY, USA: Norton.

Rubin, K. H., Fein, G., & Vanderberg, B. (1983). Play. In P. Mussen & E. M. Hetherington (Eds.), *Handbook of child psychology: Vol. 4. Socialization, personality, and social development* (pp. 693-774). New York, NY, USA: Wiley.

Santrock, J. W. (2002). *Life-Span Development*. New York, NY, USA: McGraw Hill.

Smilansky, S. (1968). *The effects of sociodramatic play on disadvantaged preschool children*. New York, NY, USA: Wiley.

Sutton-Smith, B. (2008). Play Theory: A Personal Journey and New Thoughts *American Journal of Play*, 1(1), 80-123.

Tinbergen, N. (1972). *The Animals in Its World*. Cambridge, MA, USA: Harvard University Press.

Visalberghi, A. (1958). *Esperienza e valutazione* [Experience and evaluation]. Torino, Italy: Taylor.

Vygotskij, L. S. (1976). Play and its Role in the Mental Development of the Child. In J. S. Bruner, A. Jolly, & K. Silva (Eds.), *Play. Its Role in Development and Evolution* (pp. 537-554). New York, NY, USA: Basic Books.

Winnicott, D. W. (1971). *Playing and Reality*. London, UK: Tavistock Publications.

Chapter 2 – Do children with disabilities play?

For more information on the concept of play please refer to:

Besio, S. (2017). The Need for Play for the Sake of Play. In S. Besio, D. Bulgarelli, & V. Stancheva-Popkostadinova (Eds.). *Play Development in Children with Disabilities* (pp. 9-52). Warsaw, Poland: De Gruyter Poland.

Bulgarelli, D., & Bianquin, N. (2017). Conceptual Review of Play. In S. Besio, D. Bulgarelli, & V. Stancheva-Popkostadinova (Eds.). *Play Development in Children with Disabilities* (pp. 58-70). Warsaw, Poland: De Gruyter Poland.

Vygotskij, L. S. (1976). Play and its Role in the Mental Development of the Child. In J. S. Bruner, A. Jolly, & K. Silva (Eds.), *Play. Its role in Development and Evolution* (pp. 537-554). New York, NY, USA: Basic Books.

For more information on the current concept of disability please refer to:

Bianquin N., & Bulgarelli, D. (2017). Conceptual Review of Disability. In S. Besio, D. Bulgarelli, & V. Stancheva-Popkostadinova (Eds.). *Play Development in Children with Disabilities* (pp. 71-87). Warsaw, Poland: De Gruyter Poland.

Bronfenbrenner, U. (1994). Ecological models of human development. *Readings on the Development of Children*, 2(1), 37-43.

Simeonsson, R. J., Leonardi, M., Bjorck-Akesson, E., Hollenweger, J., Lollar, D., Martinuzzi, A., & TenNapel, H. (2006). *ICF-CY: a universal tool for practice policy and research.* Document P107, Meeting of WHO Collaborating Centres for the Family of International Classifications, Tunisia.
Retrieved from http://apps.who.int/classifications/apps/icd/meetings/2006meeting/WHOFIC2006%20-%20P107%20-%20ICF-CY%20a%20universal%20tool%20for%20practice%20policy%20and%20research.pdf

World Health Organisation (2011). *World Report on Disability.* Malta: WHO. Retrieved from http://www.who.int/disabilities/world_report/2011/report.pdf

World Health Organization (2013). *How to use the ICF: A practical manual for using the International Classification of Functioning, Disability and Health (ICF).* Exposure draft for comment. Geneva, Switzerland: WHO. Retrieved from: http://www.who.int/classifications/drafticfpracticalmanual2.pdf?ua=1

For more information on the play for children with different types of disabilities please refer to:

Besio, S., Bulgarelli, D., & Stancheva-Popkostadinova, V. (Eds.) (2017). *Play Development in Children with Disabilities.* Warsaw, Poland: De Gruyter Poland.

Chapter 3 – What barriers to play do children with disabilities face?

For some studies on social environments and values and attitudes:

Frankel, F., Gorospe, C., Chang, Y., & Sugar, C. (2011). Mothers' reports of play dates and observation of school playground behavior of children having high-functioning autism spectrum disorders. *Journal of Child Psychology and Psychiatry*, 52(5), 571-579.

Lawrence, L. (2008). Hardly a walk in the park: examining disability through a mother's eyes. *Journal of Loss and trauma*, 13, 528-540.

For some studies of environmental barriers to play:

Anaby, D., Hand, C., Bradley, L., DiRezze, B., Forhan, M., DiGiacomo, A. & Law, M. (2013). The effect of the environment on participation of children and youth with disabilities: a scoping review. *Disability and Rehabilitation*, 35(19), 1589-1598.

Barron, C., Beckett, A., Coussens, M., Desoete, A., Cannon Jones, N., Lynch, H., . . . Fenney Salkeld, D. (2017). *Barriers to play and recreation for children and young people with disabilities.* Warsaw, Poland: De Gruyter Poland.

Law, M., Petrenchik, T., King, G., & Hurley, P. (2007). Perceived environmental barriers to recreational, community, and school participation for children and youth with physical disabilities. *Archives of physical medicine and rehabilitation*, 88(12), 1636-1642.

For some studies of environmental barriers to play in playgrounds:

Jeanes, R., & Magee, J. (2012). 'Can we play on the swings and rouhndabouts?': creating inclusive playspaces for disabled young people and their families. *Leisure Studies*, 31(2), 193-210.

Moore, A. & Lynch, H. (2016). Accessibility and usability of playground environments for childrern under 12: A scoping review. *Scandinavian Journal of Occupational Therapy*, 22, 331-344.

Olsen, H., & Dieser, R. (2012). "I am hoping you can point me in the right direction regarding playground accessibility": a case study of a community which lacked social policy toward playground accessibility. *World Leisure Journal*, 54(3), 269-279.

Prellwitz, M. & Tamm, M. (1999). Attitudes of key persons to accessibility problems in playgrounds for children with restricted mobility: a study in a medium-sized municipality in Northern Sweden. *Scandinavian Journal of Occupational Therapy*, 6, 166-173.

Prellwitz, M. & Skar, L. (2007). Usability of playgrounds for children with different abilities. *Occupational Therapy International*, 14(3), 144-155.

Prellwitz, M. & Skar, L. (2016). Are playgrounds a case of occupationjal injustice? Experiences of parents of children with disabilities. *Children, Youth and Environment*, 26(2), 28-42.

Ripat, J., & Becker, P. (2012). Playground usability: What do playground users say? *Occupational Therapy International*, 19, 144-153.

Yantzi, N., Young, N. & McKeever, P. (2010). The suitability of school playgrounds for physically disabled children. *Children's Geographies*, 8(1), 65-78.

For some resources and information related to policy:

Davey, C., & Lundy L. (2011). Towards greater recognition of the right to play: an analysis of Article 31 of the UNCRC. *Children & Society*, 25, 3-14.

Woolley, H. (2007). Where do the children play? How policies can influence practice. *Municipal Engineer*, 160, 89-95

Council of Europe implementation guide on participation: https://edoc.coe.int/en/youth-participation/7153-implementation-guide-to-the-child-participation-assessment-tool.html

World Health Organisation human rights-based approach to health: http://www.who.int/mediacentre/factsheets/fs323/en/

Department of Children and Youth Affairs, Ireland, Participation Hub: https://www.dcya.gov.ie/viewdoc.asp?fn=%2Fdocuments%2FPlayandRec%2F20170124ChildrenAndYoungPeopleParticipationHubMainPage.htm

See United Nations webpage for the list of General Comments related to the UNCRC: http://tbinternet.ohchr.org/_layouts/treatybodyexternal/TBSearch.aspx?Lang=en&TreatyID=5&DocTypeID=11

IPA Position Paper on the Play Rights of Children with Disabilities: http://ipaworld.org/ipa-position-statement-on-the-play-rights-of-disabled-children/

LUDI Position Statement about the Right to Play for Children with Disabilities: https://www.ludi-network.eu/wp-content/uploads/2017/11/LUDI-Position-Statement.pdf

Welsh Government (2012a). The Children and Families (Wales) Measure 2010 (Commencement No. 5). Order 2012. Cardiff, UK: Welsh Government.

Welsh Government (2012b). Play Sufficiency Assessment Toolkit. Cardiff, UK: Welsh Government.

Chapter 4 – Are our children playing?

For more information about the role of the adult in children's play:

Vygotsky, L. S. (1978). *Mind in society: The development of higher psychological processes.* Cambridge, MA, USA: Harvard University Press.

For more information on play assessment:

Besio, S., Bulgarelli, D., & Stancheva Popkostadinova, V. (2018). *Evaluation of Children's Play. Tools and Methods.* Warsaw, Poland: De Gruyter Poland.

For more information on participation:

Bourke-Taylor, H. M., Law, M., Howie, L., & Pallant, J. F. (2009). Development of the Assistance to Participate Scale (APS) for children's play and leisure activities. *Child: Care, Health and Development,* 35(5), 738-745.

Imms, C., Adair, B., Keen, D., Ullenhag, A., Rosenbaum, P., & Granlund, M. (2016). 'Participation': a systematic review of language, definitions, and constructs used in intervention research with children with disabilities. *Developmental Medicine & Child Neurology*, 58(1), 29–38.

Tools to assess playfulness:

Rogers, C. S., Impara, J. C., Frary, R. B., Harris, T., Meeks, A., Semanic-Lauth, S., & Reynolds, M. (1998). Measuring playfulness: Development of the Child Behavior Inventory of Playfulness. In M. Duncan, G. Chick, & A. Aycock (Eds.), *Play and Cultural Studies* Vol. 4, (pp. 121-135). Greenwhich, CT, USA: Ablex Publishing Corp.

Skard, G. & Bundy, A. (2008). A Test of playfulness. In D. L. Parham & L. S. Fazio (Eds.), *Play in Occupational Therapy for Children* (pp. 71-94). Amsterdam, the Netherlands: Elsevier.

Tools to assess play:

Ballard, K. D. (1981). An Observation Procedure for Assessing Children's Social Behaviours in Free Play Settings. *Educational Psychology*, 1(2), 185–99.

Ferland, F. (1997). *The Ludic Model: Play, Children with Physical Disabilities and Occupational Therapy*. Ottawa, ON, Canada: University of Ottawa Press.

Henry, A. (2008). Assessment of play and leisure in children and adolescents. In D. L. Parham & L. S. Fazio (Eds.), *Play in Occupational Therapy for Children* (pp. 95-193). Amsterdam, the Netherlands: Elsevier.

King, G., Law, M., King, S., Hurley, P., Hanna, S., Kertoy, M., Rosenbaum, P., & Young, N. (2004). *Children's Assessment of Participation and Enjoyment (CAPE) & Preferences for Activities of Children (PAC)*. San Antonio, TX, USA: Harcourt Assessment Inc.

Knox, S. (2008). Development and current use of the Revised Knox Preschool Play Scale. In D. L. Parham & L. S. Fazio (Eds.), *Play in Occupational Therapy for Children* (pp. 55-70). Amsterdam, the Netherlands: Elsevier.

Lewis, V. & Boucher, J. (1997). *Manual of the test of pretend play*. London, UK: Harcourt Brace.

McDonald, A. E., & Vigen, C. (2012). Reliability and validity of the McDonald Play Inventory. *American Journal of Occupational Therapy*, 66(4), e52–e60.

Pfeifer, L. I., Queiroz, M. A., Santos, J. L., & Stagnitti, K. E. (2011). Cross-cultural adaptation and reliability of child-initiated pretend play assessment (ChIPPA). *Canadian Journal of Occupational Therapy*, 78(3), 187-195.

Rosenblum, S., Sachs, D., & Schreuer, N. (2010). Reliability and validity of the Children's Leisure Assessment Scale. *American Journal of Occupational Therapy*, 64, 633–641.

Rubin, K. H. (2001). *The play observation scale (POS)*. College Park, MD, USA: University of Maryland.

Schneider, E. & Rosenblum, S (2014). Development, reliability and validity of My Child's Play questionnaire. *American Journal of Occupational Therapy*, 68 (3), 277-285.

Chapter 5 – How can I, as an adult, facilitate play?

Literature supporting the concept that children learn to play:

Brodin, J. (1999). Play in Children with Severe Multiple Disabilities: Play with toys – a review. *International Journal of Disability, Development and Education*, 46(1), 25-34.

Malone, D. M., & Langone, J. (1999). Teaching object-related play skills to preschool children with developmental concerns. *International Journal of Disability, Development and Education*, 46(3), 325-336.

Stagnitti, K., O'Connor, C., & Sheppard, L. (2012). Impact of Learn to Play Program on play, social competence, and language for children 5-8 who attend a specialist school. *Australian Occupational Therapy Journal*, 59, 302-311.

Literature supporting the concept that adults teach to play:

Jones, E., & Reynolds, G. (2011). *The Play's the Thing: Teachers' Roles in Children's Play* (2nd ed.). New York, NY, USA: Teachers College.

Barton, E. E., & Wolery, M. (2008). Teaching Pretend Play to Children with Disabilities: A Review of the Literature. *Topics in Early Childhood Special Education*, 28, 105-112.

Definition of scaffolding:

Wood, D., Bruner, J., & Ross, G. (1976). The role of tutoring in problem solving *Journal of Child Psychology and Psychiatry and Allied Disciplines*, 17, 89–100.

Literature supporting the right to play:

Hillman, M. (2014). Children's rights and adults' wrongs. *Children's Geographies*, 4(1), 61–67.

Besio, S., Carnesecchi, M. (2014). The Challenge of a Research Network on Play for Children with Disabilities. *Procedia-Social and Behavioral Sciences*, 146, 9-14.

Literature supporting the concept that adults is a partner in play:

Haight, W. (1998). Adult direct and indirect influences on play. In D. Bergen, D. Fromberg (Eds.), *Play from Birth to Twelve and Beyond: Contexts, Perspectives, and Meanings* (pp. 259-265). New York, NY, USA & London, UK: Garland Publishing.

Bondioli, A. (2002). *Gioco e educazione* [Play and education]. Milano, Italy: Franco Angeli.

Besio, S. (2017). The need for play for the sake of play. In S. Besio, D. Bulgarelli, V. Stancheva-Popkostadinova (Eds.), *Play Development in Children with Disabilities* (pp. 9-52). Warsaw, Poland: De Gruyter Poland.

Perino, O., & Besio, S. (2017). Mainstream Toys for Play. In S. Besio, D. Bulgarelli, V. Stancheva-Popkostadinova (Eds.), *Play Development in Children with Disabilities.* (pp. 181-200). Warsaw, Poland: De Gruyter Poland.

Literature supporting the child perspectives on play:

Spencer-Cavaliere, N., & Watkinson, E. J. (2010). Inclusion understood from the perspectives of children with disability. *Adapted Physical Activity Quarterly*, 27(4), 275-293.

Zappaterra, T., & Westling Allodi, M. (in press) *Users' Needs Report on Play for Children with Disabilities.* Warsaw, Poland: De Gruyter Poland.

Literature supporting inclusive settings:

Gupta, S. S., Henninger IV, W. R., & Vinh, M. E. (2014). *First steps to preschool inclusion: how to jumpstart your programwide plan.* Baltimore, MD, USA: Brookes Publishing.

Casper, V., & Theilheimer, R. (2010). *Introduction to early childhood education: learning together*, 1st ed. New York, NY, USA: McGraw-Hill Higher Education.

Lester, S., & Russell, W. (2010). *Children's right to play: An examination of the importance of play in the lives of children worldwide*, Working Paper No. 57. The Hague, the Netherlands: Bernard van Leer Foundation.

Chapter 6 – What Assistive Technologies exist to support play?

Definitions of Assistive Technology and Assistive Products:

World Health Organization. (2018). WHO | Global Cooperation on Assistive Technology (GATE). Retrieved from http://www.who.int/phi/implementation/assistive_technology/phi_gate/en/

ISO 9999 classification:

International Standards Organization. (2016). *ISO 9999:2016(en) Assistive products for persons with disability — Classification and terminology*. Geneva, Switzerland: ISO.

EASTIN information:

European Assistive Technology Information Network . (2016). EASTIN Brochure. Retrieved from http://www.eastin.eu/en/generalInfo/download/document-252

Literature supporting the provision of powered wheelchair for young children:

Rosen, L., Plummer, T., Sabet, A., Lange, M. L., & Livingstone, R. (2017). RESNA Position on the Application of Power Mobility Devices for Pediatric Users-Update 2017. Retrieved from http://www.resna.org/sites/default/files/legacy/Position-Papers/RESNA%20Ped%20Power%20Paper%2010_25_17%20-BOD%20approval%20Nov2_2017.pdf

Article on the use of Lego® Mindstorms® robots as manipulation tools:

Encarnação, P., Leite, T., Nunes, C., Nunes da Ponte, M., Adams, K., Cook, A., Caiado, A., Pereira, J., Piedade, G., & Ribeiro, M. (2017). Using assistive robots to promote inclusive education. *Disability and Rehabilitation: Assistive Technology*, 12(4), 352-372.

A comprehensive definition of Augmentative and Alternative Communication and further information on AAC can be found at the International Society for Augmentative and Alternative Communication (ISAAC) website https://www.isaac-online.org

United Nations Convention on the Right of Persons with Disabilities:
https://www.un.org/development/desa/disabilities/convention-on-the-rights-of-persons-with-disabilities.html

More information on the process of choosing an Assistive Product, in particular the Human Activity Assistive Technology Model:

Cook, A. M., & Polgar, J. M. (2015). *Assistive Technologies: Principles and practice*, 4th ed. St. Louis, MO, USA: Elsevier Inc.

Chapter 7 – Which toys and games are appropriate for our children?

Further reading on toys, games and playspaces:

Brougère, G. (2008). *La ronde des jeux et des jouets.* Paris, France: Editions Autrement.

Magalhães, L., & Goldstein, J. (Eds.). (2017). *Toys and communication.* London, UK: Palgrave Macmillan.

Miller Kuhaneck, H., Spitzer, S. L., & Miller, E. (2010). *Activity analysis, creativity, and playfulness in pediatric occupational therapy: Making play just right.* Sudbury, MA, USA: Jones & Bartlett.

Périno, O. (2014). *Des espaces pour jouer : pourquoi les concevoir? Comment les aménager?* Toulouse, France: Editions Erès.

Sutton Smith, B. (1986). *Toys as Culture.* New York, NY, USA: Gardner Press.

For more information on toys and Universal Design:

Anderson, K. (2005). *Universal design means toys for everyone.* Edplay magazine, Fahy-Williams Publishing Inc.

Costa, M. et al. (2007). *Juego, Juguete y discapacidad. La importancia del Diseño Universal.* Alicante, Spain: AIJU.

Costa, M., Périno. O., & Ray-Kaeser, S. (2018). *The TUET – Toys and games Usability Evaluation Tool.* Alicante, Spain: AIJU. http://www.tuet.eu

Mistrett, S., & Goetz, A. (2004). *Universal Design for Play project. Let's Play Projects.* Buffalo, NY, USA: University at Buffalo.

Chapter 9 – Which spaces are appropriate for our children?

More details on play in families and children with disabilities can be found in:

Barron, C., Beckett, A., Coussens, M., Desoete, A., Cannon Jones, N., Lynch, H., Prellwitz, M., & Fenney Salkeld, D. (2017). *Barriers to play and recreation for children and young people with disabilities.* Warsaw, Poland: De Gruyter Poland.

Buttimer, J., & Tierney, E. (2005). Patterns of leisure participation among adolescents with a mild intellectual disability. *Journal of Intellectual Disabilities,* 9(1), 25-42.

Horton, J. (2017). Disabilities, urban natures and children's outdoor play. *Social & Cultural Geography,* 18(8), 1152-1174.

Law, M., Anaby, D., Teplicky, R., Khetani, M., Coster, W., & Bedell, G. (2013). Participation in the home environment among children and youth with and without disabilities. *British Journal of Occupational Therapy,* 76(2), 58-66.

Orban, K., Ellegard, K., Thorngren-Jerneck, K., & Erlandsson, L. (2012). Shared patterns of daily occupations among parents of children aged 4-6 years old with obesity. *Journal of Occupational Science,* 19(3), 241-257.

Prellwitz, M., & Skar, L. (2006). How children with restricted mobility perceive the accessibility and usability of their home environment. *Occupational Therapy International,* 13(4), 193-206.

Rigby, P., & Gaik, S. (2007). Stability of playfulness across environmental settings: a pilot study. *Physical & Occupational Therapy in Pediatrics,* 27(1), 27-43.

More information on researching children's environments and playgrounds can be found in:

Francis, M., & Lorenzo, R. (2002). Seven realms of children's participation. *Journal of Environmental Psychology,* 22, 157-169.

Kilkelly, U., Lynch, H., O'Connell, A., Moore, A., & Field, S. (2016). *Children and the outdoors. contact with the outdoors and natural heritage among children aged 6 to 12: current trends, benefits, barriers and research requirements.* Kilkenny, Ireland: The Heritage Council.

Lynch, H., & Hayes, N. (2015). An affordance perspective on infant play in home settings: a just-right environment. *Childlinks*, 2, 17-22.

Moore, A., & Lynch, H. (2015). Accessibility and usability of playground environments for children under 12: A scoping review. *Scandanavian Journal of Occupational Therapy*, 22(5), 331-344.

Prellwitz, M., & Skar, L. (2007). Usability of playgrounds for children with different abilities. *Occupational Therapy International*, 14(3), 144-155.

Prellwitz, M., Skar, L. (2016). Are playgrounds a case of occupationjal injustice? Experiences of parents of children with disabilities. *Children, Youth and Environment*, 26(2), 28-42.

Prellwitz, M., & Tamm, M. (1999). Attitudes of key persons to accessibility problems in playgrounds for children with restricted mobility: a study in a medium-sized municipality in Northern Sweden. *Scandinavian Journal of Occupational Therapy*, 6, 166-173.

For more information on schoolyard research, namely loose parts and schoolyard greening:

Bundy, A., Wyver, S., Beetham, K., Ragen, J., Naughton, G., Tranter, P., Norman, R., Villeneuve, M., Spencer, G., Honey, A., Simpson, J., Baur, L., & Sterman, J. (2015). The Sydney Playground Project- levelling the playing field: a cluseter trial of a primary school-based intervention aiming to promote manageable risk-taking in children with disability. *BMC Public Health*, 15(1125), 1-6.

Cosco, N., Moore, R., & Smith, W. (2014). Childcare outdoor renovation as a built environment health promotion stratey: evaluating the preventing obesity by design intervention. *American Journal of Health Promotion*, 28(3), 27- 32.

Dowdell, K., Gray, T., & Malone, K. (2011). Nature and its Influence on Children's Outdoor *Play. Australian Journal of Outdoor Education*, 15, 24-35.

Kuo, F., & Faber, T. (2004). A potential natural treatment for Attention-Deficit Hyperactivity disorder: evidence from a national study. *American Journal of Public Health*, 94, 1580-1586.

See Rick Hansen Foundation guidelines for creating accessible playspaces in schools: https://www.rickhansen.com/Portals/2/Documents/PAC%20toolkit_7JUN11.pdf

See Learning Through Landscapes, UK, for school support and programmes related to outdoor learning: http://www.ltl.org.uk/about/about-ltl.php

See Evergreen Canada for links to greening school grounds: http://www.evergreen.ca/our-impact/children/greening-school-grounds/

See also Children, Youth and Environments, (2014), volume 24, no 2 for an entire issue on green school environments

For more information on designing playspaces and Universal Design:

Design for play for communities, from Play Scotland/England: http://www.playscotland.org/wp-content/uploads/Design-for-Play-a-guide-to-creating-successful-place-spaces.pdf

Places for play and play value: http://www.freeplaynetwork.org.uk/pubs/PfP2.pdf

Goltsman, S. (2011). Outdoor play settings: an inclusive approach. In W. Preiser and K. Smith (Eds.), *Universal Design Handbook*. London, UK: McGraw-Hill.

PlayCore & Utah State University. (2010). *Me2: 7 principles of inclusive playground design*. Chattanooga, TN, USA, TN: Playcore.

Rick Hansen Foundation for some ideas about designing for inclusive play: https://www.rickhansen.com/Our-Work/School-Program/Accessible-Play-Spaces

For more information on the Playground Audit Tool, please refer to www.ludi-network.eu or the CEUD/National Disability Authority Ireland: http://universaldesign.ie/News-events/News/NDA-Research-Promotion-Scheme-Universal-Design-2017-Award-of-Funding.html

For more information on enabling play:

Child in the City - information on the Playing Out initiative: https://www.childinthecity.org/2017/11/28/bbc-video-on-playing-out-receives-8-million-views/

Google Images for ideas and pictures: https://www.google.ie/search?q=designing+outdoor+play+at+home+for+children+with+disabilities&rlz=1C1KMZB_enIE576IE579&source=lnms&tbm=isch&sa=X&ved=0ahUKEwjMorPx2bnYAhVoB8AKHV03BbAQ_AUICigB&biw=667&bih=635

Maketime2Play: http://www.maketime2play.co.uk/play-chat/further-reading/

Rigby, P., & Huggins, L. (2003). Enabling young children to play by creating supportive environments. In L. Letts, P. Rigby & D. Stewart (Eds.), *Using Environments to Enable Occupational Performance* (pp. 153-174). Thorofare, NJ, USA: Slack Inc.

Sample ideas for designing autism-friendly environments: http://shineireland.com/the-autism-friendly-environment/

Example of a local airport addressing autism-friendly environments: https://www.bristolairport.co.uk/at-the-airport/special-assistance/other-advice

Sense Play Inquiry, UK: https://www.youtube.com/playlist?list=PL3cz6p9Us2bP6NIaZ47OzO48fQnMBFXnw

Appendix

Outdoor Play and Social Inclusion: Public Playspace Audit Version 5, 2017

Helen Lynch, Alice Moore and Maria Prellwitz

Outdoor Play and Social Inclusion: Public Playspace Audit RECORD FORM

Playspace Information

Location: ____________________

Date of Assessment (dd/mm/yyyy): ____________________

Time of Assessment: ____________________

Weather on the day of Assessment: ____________________

Observer (Name and Discipline): ____________________

Purpose of Audit

For what purpose was the Audit tool being used?

	Yes	No
To assess the design of an existing playspace		
To assess for the re-design of an existing playspace		
To observe a child in an existing playspace		
To plan for the design of a new playspace		

Playspace Information

Playspace Type

Public Playspace (e.g. playground) .... ☐ Other .... ☐

Private Playspace (e.g. school)................ ☐ If other, please specify:

Hospital Playspace.................................. ☐ ____________________

Observation Information

This section is only applicable if the purpose of the Audit was to observe a child in an existing playspace

Name: ____

Gender: ____________________

Primary means of mobility		**Primary means of communication**	
Walks independently	☐	Verbal	☐
Walks with assistance	☐	Written / Pictorial	☐
Uses crutches/ walker	☐	Sign	☐
Wheelchair (manual)	☐	Gesture / Body movements	☐
Wheelchair (electric)	☐	Communication Board	☐
Other (specify): ______		Computer / electronic	☐

Conditions that may affect child participation and/ or performance in play

Name of Condition: ______________________________

Tick all that apply

	Intellectual	*Physical*	*Speech or Language*	*Sensory*	*Emotional/ Behavioural/ Attention*	*Other*
Social Play						
Physical Play						
Sensory Play						
Communication						
Cognitive						

Comments: ______________________________

____

____

____

____

____

____

____

____

LYNCH, MOORE, PRELLWITZ VERSION 5: 2017:
contact h.lynch@ucc.ie for further information on the development of this tool

Public Playspace Audit

Section 1: General Information

Date (dd/mm/yyyy):

Time:

Weather:

Observer:

For what reason is the playspace audit tool being used

	Yes	No	To some extent	Description
To assess the design of an existing plays-pace				
To assess for the re-design of an exist-ing playspace				
To observe a child in an existing playspace				
To plan for the design of a new playspace				

Finding out about the playspace				
	Yes	No	To some extent	Description
Is the information about the playspace, including information about the play opportunities, and directions, available (is information available online; are photos and comments available; information available by phone)?				
Is the playspace listed on the County Council information site?				

Section 2: Location and General Site Information				
	Yes	No	To some extent	Description (text and pictures where applicable)
Transport / Parking				
Are there accessible routes to the playspace by foot, car, and/ or public transport?				
Are there parking spaces next to the playspace or close by?				
Are there allocated accessible parking spaces available?				
Is there a reasonable distance from car parking facilities to the playspace?				

Getting into the playspace				
Are walking routes to playspace accessible (smooth surfaces; wide paths; gentle slopes; safe crossing points with dropped kerbs)?				
Is the playspace easy to get into (if there is a gate, is it easy to operate)?				
Is the playspace welcoming?				
Is it aesthetically pleasing?				

Navigating arround the playspace				
Does the colour combination avoid the use of (orange/brown), (blue/ green) and (red/ green) [please note that these colour combinations should be avoided for persons that are colour-blind]				
Is text kept to a minimum and easy to read with Braille, symbols/ pictorial images as well as text?				

Is signage located at wheelchair or child friendly height (i.e. 1m from ground)				
Is there a map that shows users how to move around the space and where all items are located?				

Toileting and changing facilities				
Are there accessible toilets on site or nearby?				
Are there accessible changing facilities located nearby?				

General maintenance				
Is the playspace clean?				
Are there litter bins available?				
Is the playspace appropriately maintained?				
Is there contact information for maintenance of the play area?				

Section 3: Internal Accessibility and Usability of the Playspace				
	Yes	No	To some extent	Description (text and pictures where applicable)
Seating				
Is it adjacent to play equipment?				
Do some seats have arm and backrests?				
Can visitors using mobility devices, including wheelchairs sit between other people without blocking a path or feeling like an after-thought?				
Does the seating bench have a wide level space beside it for wheelchair or buggies to be placed alongside?				
Tables				
Can children and adults using mobility devices, including wheelchairs use tables provided – i.e. are there tables high enough for people's legs to go under the table?				

Access aids				
Are there access aids present e.g. ramps, transfer points, ropes, handrails				
Is the highest point in the playground accessible to all users?				
Can the highest point in the playground be accessed by various means (stairs, ramps, ropes, etc.)?				
Do the access aids meet advised requirements e.g. ramps, transfer points, ropes, handrails?				
Are stairs and ramps contrast marked before and after?				

Pathway and circulation				
Does the playspace incorporate an intuitive flow and looping between play components that results in repetitive and creative play?				

Is there adequate space for movement throughout the play environment for users with assistive devices and/ or those who require personal assistance?				
Are surfacing and the main pathway through the play area accessible so that all individuals have an equitable way to access and travel throughout the play environment?				
Are there grassy and gravelly surfaces for variety?				
Are there shrubs and perennials with bushy growth placed adjacent walking surfaces? (Please note that shrubs and perennials with bushy growth should be avoided ad-jacent walking surfaces)				

Are there trees with shallow roots placed near walking surfaces? (Please note that trees with shallow roots should not be placed near walking surfaces as they easily break up the soil)				
Location & landscaping				
Does the design of play area fit within its location?				
Is the noise level comfortable?				
Does the playspace incorporate varied surfaces: open and flat; mounding; planting?				
Sun/ Shade Balance – Are there any shaded areas e.g. provided by canopies, sails, trees or other type of shade structures?				

Wind/ Rain Balance – Are there any covered areas e.g. provided by canopies, sails, or other type of shelter structures?				
Can the playspace be used during all seasons of the year?				
Safety				
Are there opportunities for risk and challenge along with a balance of a reasonable need for safety?				
Does the playspace incorporate varied ways of ensuring safety in a creative way (e.g. boundaries that are creative and not just fences; for example, mounding and vegetation ton create a sense of enclosure)?				
Are accessible, comfortable supervision areas available that offer clear views of the play area for parents or caregivers with and without disabilities?				

Has unnecessary risk been eliminated? Does the play area look necessarily safe?				
Are appropriate fall zones provided under elevated play equip-ment?				

Section 4: General Design				
	Yes	No	To some extent	Description (text and pictures where applicable)
Age and ability				
Does the playspace allow for children of different ages to play together?				
Does the playspace incorporate graduated levels of challenge?				
Does the playspace allow for intergenerational play to occur?				
Has due consideration been given to children with a range of physical, sensory, cognitive, communication, social disabilities/abilities including age and size and their use of and inclusion in the playspace? (including variety for developmental abilities and need for challenges)				

Nature				
Are there opportunities for children to play with nature and natural elements (e.g. wild flowers, trees, long grass)?				
Is the planting toxic or thorny? (Please note that toxic and thorny plants should not be used)				
Is the planting strong smelling? (Please note that flowers with a strong fragrance should be avoided as well as plants that can disperse lots of pollen with the wind)				

Section 5: Play Affordances in the Playspace				
	Yes	No	To some extent	Description (text and pictures where applicable)
Social play				
Group or cooperative play opportunities – is there space for group games, sports activities that can be accessed by all?				
Are there opportunities to help others or to support others?				
Are there peaceful play opportunities to play alone or in groups, private spaces to play or hide, hidey holes, nooks and crannies, tunnels, cosy spaces?				
Is the play environment usable by individuals with diverse abilities creating an atmosphere of mutual respect and acceptance to foster friendships and understanding?				

LYNCH, MOORE, PRELLWITZ VERSION 5: 2017:
contact h.lynch@ucc.ie for further information on the development of this tool

Physical play				
Does the playspace allow for: running, crawling, jumping, rocking, swinging, sliding, hanging, climbing, spinning, balancing, and bouncing?				
Does the playspace allow for whole body movements including manipulation- loose parts, at a variety of heights- e.g. water/ sand/ twisting games?				

Sensory play				
Is there access to natural materials; twigs, logs, boulders, sticks? Are there accessible places to play around natural areas?				
Are there opportunities to explore sight/ visual experiences (e.g. textures and shapes, reflected light, strong colour/ contrast, pattern)?				

Are there opportunities to explore sound experiences (movement and switch activated by using small or large motor movements- e.g. playing with water-sound makers or instruments)?				
Are there opportunities to explore scent (e.g. planting)?				
Are there opportunities to explore tactile experiences (e.g. carvings, range of materials sand water, loose parts, range of surface textures and materials)?				
Are there opportunities to explore movement and balance: Exploring balance, coordination, strength, spatial awareness and dynamic movement?				

Communication				
Are there opportunities to socialise with peers?				
Are there opportunities to socialise with adults?				
Do children have opportunities to have a say and negotiate?				
Do children have opportunities to share ideas and feelings with others?				
Are children consulted on equipment in the playspace and the design of the playspace?				

Cognitive				
Is there open space for imaginative games together e.g. without equipment for play-ground games/drama?				
Does the playspace incorporate a variety of shapes and colours?				
Are there multiple op-portunities for children to learn/ practice skills?				
Do children have a choice of activities that they can determine whether or not they want to participate in?				
Are there opportunities for children to develop spatial awareness and planning skills?				

Additional comments:

Outdoor Play and Social Inclusion: Public Playspace Audit

SUMMARY FORM

	Good design features (provide pictures and text)	**Poor design features** (provide pictures and text)	**Recommenda-tions** (provide pictures and text)
Section 1: General Infor-mation			
Section 2: Location and General Site Information			
Section 3: Internal Ac-cessibility and Usability of the Playspace			
Section 4: General Design			
Section 5: Play Affordances in the Playspace			

LYNCH, MOORE, PRELLWITZ VERSION 5: 2017:
contact h.lynch@ucc.ie for further information on the development of this tool

The Following resources were used to guide the development of this *"Outdoor Play & Social Inclusion: Public Playspace Audit"*

1. Play for all: Providing Play Facilities for disabled Children
http://www.dessa.ie/sites/default/files/files/Play%20for%20All.pdf

2. Access Inside Out: A Guide to Making Community Facilities Accessible
http://www.dessa.ie/sites/default/files/files/Access%20Inside%20Out.pdf

3. Design for Play: A guide to creating successful playspaces
http://www.playengland.org.uk/media/70684/design-for-play.pdf

4. Me2: 7 Principles of Inclusive Playground Design
Book available on request from Playcore

5. Developing Accessible Playspace: A Good Practice Guide
http://ibrarian.net/navon/paper/Developing_accessible_play_space__a_good_practice.pdf?paperid=3017456

6. Space for active play: Developing child-inspired playspace for older children
http://spotidoc.com/doc/75231/space-for-active-play---developing-child-inspired

7. Can Play Will Play
http://www.fieldsintrust.org/Upload/Documents/Products/can_play_will_play_1004006374.pdf

8. Let's Play: Creating accessible playspaces a toolkit for school-based groups
https://www.rickhansen.com/Portals/2/Documents/PAC%20toolkit_7JUN11.pdf

9. The Good Playspace Guide: I Can Play Too
http://www.fairplayforchildren.org/pdf/1224539481.pdf

10. Designing for all children
https://www.whitehutchinson.com/children/articles/designforall.shtml

11. Playspace design: A higher level of inclusive play
https://issuu.com/penchura/docs/higher_level_of_inclusive_play

12. The principles for inclusive play
http://touchedbyolivia.com.au/inclusiveplayspace/

13. Inclusive play design guide
https://www.accessibleplayground.net/wp-content/uploads/2016/05/Inclusive-Play-Design-Guide-LowRes-2.pdf

14. Everybody plays (Universal Playground Design)
http://www.google.ie/url?sa=t&rct=j&q=&esrc=s&source=web&cd=54&ved=0ahUKEwj60KTg2avKAhXD-A4KHTRKDlw4MhAWCC4wAw&url=http%3A%2F%2Focalafl.iqm2.com%2FCitizens%2FFileOpen.aspx%3FType%3D4%26ID%3D1491&usg=AFQjCNE6aR2p_WwwzEP-EnEFrFLJ4MUnKA

15. Researching children's designs for a child friendly playspace at Rouse Hill town centre
https://www.westernsydney.edu.au/__data/assets/pdf_file/0005/713651/Researching_Childrens_Designs_for_a_Child_Friendly_Play_Space_at_Rouse_Hill_Town_Centre.pdf

16. Hume Playspace Planning Framework and Reference Guide
http://www.hume.vic.gov.au/files/sharedassets/hume_website/publications/strategies_and_plans/playspace_planning_framework_and_reference_guide.pdf

17. Playspaces: Planning and design
http://www.playwales.org.uk/login/uploaded/documents/INFORMATION%20SHEETS/play%20spaces%20-%20planning%20and%20design.pdf

18. An informational guide to young children's outdoor playspaces 7Cs
http://www.wstcoast.org/playspaces/outsidecriteria/7Cs.pdf

19. Move more North Carolina: A guide to creating active outdoor playspaces
http://www.eatsmartmovemorenc.com/ActivePlaySpaces/Texts/PlaySpacesGuide-HiRez.pdf

20. Planning for play in a playground
http://www.planforplay.org/planning_for_play/design_approach.php

21. Playground accessibility: ADA Compliance
http://www.ucdenver.edu/academics/colleges/medicalschool/programs/atp/Documents/Playground%20Accessibility.pdf

22. Inclusive play
http://www.keroul.qc.ca/DATA/PRATIQUEDOCUMENT/262_fr.pdf

23. Design guidance for playspaces
http://www.forestry.gov.uk/pdf/fce-design-guidance-for-play-spaces.pdf/$FILE/fce-design-guidance-for-play-spaces.pdf

24. Design principles for nature playspaces in nature centres and other natural areas
http://www.greenheartsinc.org/uploads/Green_Hearts_Design_Principles_for_Nature_Play_Spaces.pdf

25. Developing and Managing Playspaces
http://www.playwales.org.uk/login/uploaded/documents/Publications/Community%20Toolkit%202016.pdf

Bei Fragen zur Produktsicherheit wenden Sie sich bitte an:
If you have any questions regarding product safety,
please contact:

Walter de Gruyter GmbH
Genthiner Straße 13
10785 Berlin
productsafety@degruyterbrill.com